Alternative Treatments for Cancer

Steven Lehrer, M.D.

Nelson-Hall nh Chicago

for Pamela

I wish to express my gratitude to Dr. Bernard Roswit, whose lectures on cancer and cancer therapy suggested the subject matter for this book. I also wish to thank Pamela Dunn Lehrer and Dr. Herbert Rosenthal for their timely support and encouragement.

Lehrer, Steven.
   Alternative treatments for cancer.

   Bibliography: p.
   Includes index.
   1. Cancer. I. Title. [DNLM: 1. Neoplasms—
Therapy. QZ266 L522a]
   RC263.L367   616.9′94   78–31430
   ISBN 0-88229-473-3 (cloth)
   ISBN 0-88229-666-3 (paper)

Contents

Introduction   v
1   The Cancer Problem   1
2   Breast Cancer   13
3   Lung Cancer   23
4   Cancer of the Female Reproductive Organs   31
5   Cancer of the Digestive Tract   47
6   Cancer of the Male Genital Tract and Urinary Tract   69
7   Skin Cancer   79
8   Leukemias and Lymphomas   85
9   Tumors of the Nervous System   103
10   Tumors of the Eye   111
11   Tumors of the Head and Neck   113
12   Tumors of Bone and Soft Tissue   131
13   Tumors of Children   137
14   Tumors of the Thyroid and Adrenal Glands   143
15   Cancer and Baloney:
     Management Methods of Dubious Value   151
16   In Brief   173
     Bibliography   175
     Index   180

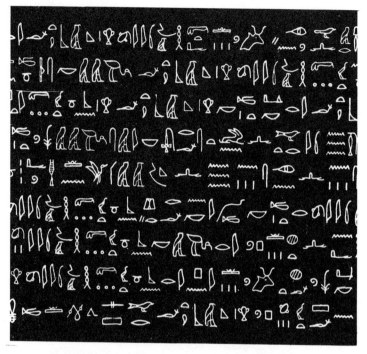

Hieroglyphic transliteration of a portion of the
Edwin Smith Surgical Papyrus (ca. 1700 B.C.),
which probably contains the first mention of
breast tumors in history. The hieroglyphs describe
case number 45: "Bulging Tumors of the Breast."
According to the papyrus "there is no treatment.
If thou findest bulging tumors in any member of a
man thou shalt treat him according to these
directions" (in other words, by omitting
treatment).

From J. H. Breasted, *The Edwin Smith Surgical Papyrus*. Published for the New York Historical Society by the University of Chicago Press, 1930, p. 405 and plate XVI. Courtesy of the New York Historical Society and the American Cancer Society.

Introduction

Cancer. Malignancy. Tumor.

These are words that cause most people to freeze with fear. Many persons with obvious symptoms of cancer will not visit a physician until the eleventh hour, such is their anxiety. Still others will accept without question any treatment, no matter how drastic, that the doctor prescribes for a tumor. For, they reason, isn't anything better than death from cancer?

Consider these situations:

A thirty-eight-year-old secretary finds a cancer in her breast. Her doctor performs a radical mastectomy. Subsequently, her husband sues for divorce, not wanting to be married to a woman with one breast. An alternative to mastectomy could have saved her breast and maybe her marriage as well.

A forty-year-old man has a cancer of his tongue. His doctor tells him that most of his tongue must be cut out. After the operation, the man can no longer talk, slobbers, swallows with difficulty, and cannot go back to work. A less mutilating alternative would have saved his tongue.

A forty-five-year-old man finds that he has a tumor on a vocal cord. The treatment results in the loss of his larynx, loss of normal speech, and a hole in his neck to breathe through for the rest of his life. Another form of treatment might have stopped the cancer without these disabling physical changes.

A forty-four-year-old insurance executive notices blood in his stool one day and discovers he has rectal cancer. Surgery is performed without delay. The man is cured, but he must cope with a colostomy for life. This executive could have been cured in another way so that a colostomy was not needed.

A fifty-five-year-old man with an active sex life has a routine physical and discovers he has cancer of the prostate. After surgery the man is impotent. A different form of treatment could have been used to cure him and preserve his potency.

Sadly, many patients are not aware of what cancer treatment will do to their body functions. And they frequently do not know that, for the cancers listed above as well as for other forms of cancer, there are nondisfiguring treatments that may be as good as the drastic, old, well-accepted ones. So they don't ask.

And even when asked, some doctors are reluctant to deviate from the old standard therapies unless the patient refuses them outright. Other doctors are unaware that alternatives in cancer therapy even exist.

Therefore the medical consumer must be aware of what is possible in cancer therapy, as well as what is not. For the patient, not the doctor, must be the one capable of adjusting to body changes after cancer therapy.

This book, then, is a consumer's guide to cancer and cancer therapy. All of the alternatives can be found here.

1 The Cancer Problem

Cancer is on the rise. As infectious diseases such as pneumonia are brought under control with antibiotics and other new drugs, people live longer and the cancer incidence increases. In the United States today, deaths from cancer are exceeded only by deaths from heart or kidney disease. One person in four will have cancer during his lifetime. Three hundred thousand Americans will die from cancer this year. Why do they get cancer?

In spite of the billions of dollars that have been spent on research, the cause of cancer, as well as its cure, elude us. We know that there are chemical and structural differences between the normal cell and the cancer cell, but their exact significance remains unclear.

Cancer is widespread throughout the vegetable and animal kingdoms. Plant cancers occur in clover, sunflowers, and other common plants. Cancer of the breast develops in dogs, anal cancer occurs in gray horses, and cancer of the eyelid afflicts cattle. Cancer occurs with great frequency in mice, making these rodents quite valuable for the study of transplantable cancers.

Racial and environmental factors may have some bearing on the cause of human cancer. Cancer of the inner nasal cavity, the nasopharynx, is unusually frequent in Chinese people. Cancer of the liver occurs many times more often in Malay groups and West African Bantu than in Caucasian peoples. Kaposi's hemorrhagic sarcoma, a rare form of skin cancer, almost exclusively afflicts Chinese, Jews, and the Bantu peoples of the Mediterranean basin. Malignant melanoma, a tumor that develops from skin moles, rarely occurs in African negroes, but it is more common in American blacks with a white racial heritage. Cancer of the stomach develops twice as frequently in the Japanese and Icelanders as in other peoples and is seen an average of ten years earlier in Japanese than in Caucasians. Cancer of the uterine cervix is extremely rare in Jewish women but quite commonplace among Puerto Ricans and blacks.

Until the 1950s, physicians commonly assumed that the preponderance of certain cancers among specific peoples was entirely due to racial transmission. Careful surveys since then, however, have revealed extrinsic causes in some cases. The frequency of stomach cancer in Iceland may be due to cancer-inducing hydrocarbons in the smoke that Icelanders use to cure fish and meats. Cancer of the liver may be so common among the Bantu partly because of their severe nutritional deficiencies, for the incidence of the disease drops sharply when the Bantu start eating a nutritionally adequate diet.

The frequency of cancer occurrence is slightly greater in women than in men, due to the great susceptibility of the uterus and the breast to malignancy. But the incidence of cancers of certain other regions of the body also differs between the sexes, and this is difficult to explain. Why, for example, should most stomach cancer occur in men? Why should most oral cancer affect men? Why is most thyroid cancer seen in women? No one knows.

In addition, people of different ages are likely to have different forms of cancer. The disease is generally one of middle and old age. But retinoblastoma, an eye tumor; Wilms' tumor of the kidney; and neuroblastoma, a nerve tumor, affect children almost exclusively. Cancer of the testicle is a disease of young males, usually under the age of thirty. Carcinomas of the breast and uterus have their greatest incidence in women between the ages of forty-five to sixty-five and decrease in relative frequency thereafter. Some cancers, such as those of fibrous tissue, are exceptions to the age distribution patterns and occur at the same rate throughout life.

The most intensive studies on the cause of cancer are being focused on viruses. Numerous animal cancers have been shown to be produced by viruses. Electron microscopic studies have revealed viruslike particles in cells from human leukemia patients, breast cancers, and rectal cancers. One human cancer found in Africa, the Burkitt tumor, almost certainly is of viral origin; unfortunately, the virus responsible has not yet been positively isolated and identified. And we don't know why some animals exposed to the virus do not get cancer.

Another factor that appears to play a role in the development of cancer is heredity. Scientists have demonstrated this factor in animals through selective breeding, particularly inbreeding, to develop strains of mice in which different types of cancer appear consistently in each generation. In humans, similar genetic tendencies can be followed through families. A perfect example of this situation is the mothers, daughters, and granddaughters in certain families who acquire cancer of the breast. In other families, cancer of the stomach is a common disease. This familial distribution has occurred too frequently to be considered coincidental, and conclusions about the role of heredity are supported by reports of cancers of similar type and regional distribution in identical twins. Perhaps a child may inherit the type of stomach or breast in which cancer is most prone to occur rather than inheriting the disease itself.

As a rule, two factors must be present for heredity to bring on human cancer: (1) the genetic background susceptibility, which is not the same for every variety of cancer, and (2) an inciting or causal factor that precipitates the onset of the cancer in the predisposed tissue. Occasionally, through chance breeding in which the genetic factors are magnified, the hereditary tendency becomes manifest. This is shown in an inherited condition of the skin, xeroderma pigmentosum, which results in the loss of all protection from the irritating rays of the sun.

Portions of the skin exposed to sunlight, notably on the hands and face, inevitably develop multiple lethal cancers. The only way for people with xeroderma pigmentosum to avoid cancer is to avoid sunlight.

And there is one form of cancer in which heredity is without a doubt practically the only causative factor involved. This is retinoblastoma, the previously mentioned eye tumor, which is the second most common malignant tumor of childhood. Occurring once every twenty thousand births, retinoblastoma can be seen as a white mass filling an infant's eye. Before the advent of modern cancer therapy, physicians knew only that 6 percent of all cases of retinoblastoma ran in families.

But within the last few years, surgery, high-energy radiation therapy, and chemotherapy have made cure and long-term survival after retinoblastoma a reality in many cases. Survivors of this cancer have been observed to transmit the disease to their offspring 50 percent of the time if retinoblastoma runs in their family. This pattern of inheritance, known as autosomal dominance, was first observed by a monk, Gregor Mendel, in his genetic experiments with garden peas over one hundred years ago.

A third factor, recently experimentally demonstrated to have an intriguing effect on the development of cancer, is the result of chronic psychic stress. Doctors have seen many instances of cancer that have occurred after the loss of a loved one and the concomitant feelings of hopelessness and despair. Other researchers have observed a high cancer incidence in people who tend to repress their emotions while leading a life characterized by endurance and order.

Dr. Vernon Riley, chairman of the Department of Microbiology at the Pacific Northwest Research Foundation in Seattle, reports in the August 8, 1975, issue of *Science* on his recent experiments using stress to induce breast cancer in mice. Female infant mice carrying the Bittner mammary tumor virus—an organism that can induce breast tumors in animals—were divided into groups and subjected to various degrees of stress. Chronic anxiety was induced in some of the animals by daily experimental manipulation and exposure to dust, odor, noise, aerosols, and noxious chemical agents. Those mice that were stressed had a significantly higher incidence of breast cancer than nonstressed mice.

Physical trauma, sometimes a single blow, can lead to the development of cancer. Extensive burn scars are prone to develop cancer within themselves after a period of years. The pressure of hot pipestems and ill-fitting dentures may cause cancer of the lip or gums.

Chemical trauma is also a factor related to cancer. An excellent example of cancer that arises from chronic chemical irritation is that which occurs in the cheeks of Hindus who are addicted to chewing a mixture of areca nut, betel nut, and lime. Chewing plain tobacco, by the way, has the same end result. And everyone knows the hazards of smoking cigarettes.

A person's occupation may involve elements leading to cancer. In the early 1960s many organic and inorganic compounds used in manufacturing and other processes were recognized to be carcinogenic agents, that is, capable of producing cancers. The amount of agent required to produce cancer may be so minute that it causes no apparent irritation at the time of exposure, yet continued contact gradually produces tissue changes that ultimately become cancerous. The precancerous change may be so permanent that a malignant tumor will develop many years after an occupation has been abandoned.

The compound vinyl chloride, a component of some plastics, has most recently been implicated in the development of liver cancer. Workers in the dyestuffs industry who are exposed to the chemicals aniline, benzidine, or beta-napthylamine may later suffer from cancer of the urinary bladder. Cancer of the lung and respiratory tract occur in workers who inhale chrome salts, asbestos dust, or nickel carbonyl. Leukemia sometimes affects persons exposed to benzene. Contact with coal tar, crude mineral oils, crude paraffins, pitch, and arsenical compounds occasionally results in multiple cancers of the skin. Prior to the mid

1920s, painters applying radium numerals on watches ingested the radioactive substance by moistening the brush tip on their tongues; these unfortunate people later contracted bone cancer. Such hazardous manufacturing processes were halted after the danger was discovered.

Too much occupational radiation may lead to cancer. Radiologists and X-ray technicians, dentists who use X rays without shielding themselves completely, orthopedic surgeons who overuse fluoroscopy for setting fractures—all these workers have a high incidence of leukemia compared to the general population. Too much exposure of the hands leads to radiation dermatitis and ultimately cancer. Many distinguished radiologists in the past died from the effects of the radiation they received.

Certain diseases have long been recognized as factors leading to cancer. Malignant tumors do not develop inevitably, but they occur with such frequency that the term precancerous has been applied to these precursor diseases.

One precancerous condition is the presence of gallstones. The incidence of cancer of the gallbladder is approximately 5 percent of the general population. But 98 percent of the persons who develop this cancer have or have had gallstones, a strong indication that the chronic irritation of the stones is a causative factor of the cancer.

Leukoplakia, another example of a precancerous condition, is a disease in which thick, white patches appear on the mucous membranes of the tongue, lip, cheek, floor of the mouth, palate, or tonsil. Especially susceptible to this disorder are smokers; leukoplakia in the mouth of a pipe enthusiast is frequently called a smoker's patch. Cancer develops with some frequency in these patches of preexisting leukoplakia.

Syphilis of the tongue sometimes predisposes to the development of cancer in this organ. The "glass tongue," so called because of its characteristic appearance, is the only part of the body afflicted by syphilis that is made vulnerable to cancer by this disease.

The neck of the womb (cervix uteri) may subsequently become cancerous if badly scarred, eroded, or chronically infected, as sometimes occurs after childbirth. Certain benign tumors are precancerous in varying percentages: polyps of the colon, papillomas of the urinary bladder, and pigmented moles of the skin.

Because of the widly diverse elements that figure in causing cancer, a "multiple-step induction theory" has been proposed, which states that numerous factors such as chemical exposure or radiation exposure can alter immunity and body defenses, leading to cancer. This theory is supported by the fact that immunity is known to be depressed in many forms of cancer. Yet the theory has weaknesses.

Any good theory should allow a scientist to make predictions. The multiple-step induction theory does not do this. So most advances in cancer diagnosis and therapy are still being made by trial and error. Close observation of cancer cells themselves furnishes some of the most relevant clues.

The control center of a cell is located within its nucleus, a central package of the compound deoxyribonucleic acid, or DNA for short. All heredity is transferred from generation to generation through the composition of the DNA.

In a cancer cell, the DNA molecules are seen to be disorganized. During replication of a normal human cell, the DNA is contained in forty-six distinct units called chromosomes, which can be seen with an ordinary microscope. A replicating cancer cell frequently contains more than the normal number of chromosomes. In one form of leukemia, a specific abnormal chromosome may be found. As can be expected, chemical processes in the cell, all controlled by the DNA, are markedly altered in cancer.

The chemical structure of all cellular protein molecules is encoded within the DNA, and cells are constantly synthesizing proteins. Cancer cells can sometimes first be identified by the abnormal proteins they produce. For example, the cells of multiple myeloma, a bone marrow cancer, make Bence-Jones protein, first detected in the urine of myeloma patients more than a hundred years ago.

Oxygen consumption and tissue acidity are altered in cancer cells. The metabolism of sugar is speeded up. Normal cells cannot survive or reproduce without oxygen, but malignant cells can. Cellular enzyme activity heightens as normal cells are displaced by malignant ones.

Ordinarily, cells will not displace one another. In laboratory single-layer cell cultures, a normal cell will lose movement when another normal cell is contacted, a phenomenon known as contact inhibition. Cancer cells have independent movement. Contact inhibition is lost. And as the masses of cancer cells accumulate, another strange growth takes place.

Groups of cancer cells are capable of causing new blood vessel formation to nourish them. Like little roads built from busy main highways, these new arteries and veins branch off from normal vessels. Researchers believe that the malignant tissue must elaborate some substance that stimulates new vessel formation; whatever it may be, this substance has never been isolated and identified.

The cancer cell's disagreeable ability to displace normal cells and carry a blood supply with it allows this unwelcome invader to enter vital organs. Entrance into contiguous tissue may occur by metastasis. The metastatic cancer cell breaks off from the original lesion and is carried by the blood and lymph systems to distant parts of the body, where it sets up shop—though the rate of growth in the new location is wholly unpredictable.

In general, cancer cells divide at a higher rate than do normal cells, but this is not always true. For example, in the organization of a callus in a fractured bone and in the relining of the uterus by surface cells after menstruation, the normal cells divide at a higher rate than do cancer cells. Also, malignant tumors have intermittent growth and latent periods. A case in point is breast cancer: the first distant metastasis may not develop until ten years after the original breast tumor had been removed.

What was that distant tumor cell doing for ten years? Why didn't it start growing before? No one knows. We only know for certain that each type of cancer behaves in its own way.

There are basically two types of cancer, according to the simplest method of classification: carcinoma and sarcoma. Carcinoma usually originates in epithelial tissue, such as skin; sarcoma develops from connective tissue, such as bone or cartilage. But actually, there are as many varieties of cancer as there are organs and tissues within the body. Each type and subtype of cancer has its own special appearance and can be identified with an ordinary microscope.

Cancer may be classified according to the stage of the disea̅e. Examples are: (1) early or localized cancer, still confined to the tissue of origin and frequently curable; (2) metastatic cancer, spread to lymph nodes or invading contiguous structures; and (3) cancer widely disseminated throughout the body.

A third classfication of cancer is by grading into one of four degrees of malignancy as determined by microscopic examination. Grade one cancers (barely malignant) tend to re̅emble the cells of the tissue from which they originated; a grade one thyroid cancer, for example, that has spread to the lung still looks like thyroid tissue. Highly malignant grade four cancers are composed of very actively dividing cells and look very unlike the tissue from which they were derived. Grade two and three cancers represent intermediate degrees of differentiation and reproduction. Usually grade four cancers grow more rapidly, metastasize earlier and more widely, pursue a more rapid course, and have a lower rate of curability than the other three grades.

Certain prefixes are usually added to the basic designations of carcinoma and sarcoma to indicate the tissue of origin. For example, a sarcoma originating in bone and tending to produce bony (osseous) tissue is called an osteogenic sarcoma. A fibrosarcoma begins in fibrous (connective) tissue. The prefix *adeno* connotes the presence of ductal or glandular elements in the tumor, as in adenocarcinoma of the stomach. Cancers of the epithelial cells, which form the skin and certain mucous membranes, may be termed epidermoid carcinomas. A primary cancer is one that has originated in the tissue in question.

For reasons that remain mysterious, the incidence of various forms of cancer is changing. For example, cancer of the stomach has decreased in frequency by 63 percent in the last twenty-five years. Many busy family doctors have not seen a stomach cancer in years.

Yet lung cancer has increased drastically in the last twenty years, up 125 percent. And more women are now getting lung tumors, a disease that was once almost entirely restricted to men. Larger numbers of female smokers, the "You've come a long way, baby!" phenomenon, may explain why more women are affected, but no one knows why the total number has ballooned so drastically.

In spite of the changing incidence, however, more people are surviving cancer today than ever before. Overall cure rates for some cancers are up, especially prostate, uterus, thyroid, kidney, bladder, larynx, skin melanoma, Hodgkin's disease (a cancer of the lymphatic system), and leukemia. Progress is significant: twenty-five years ago, one patient in four was cured. Today one in three is saved, a remarkable gain at current rates of cancer incidence.

There are three reasons why we are saving more cancer victims. More cancers are being diagnosed early because of greater public awareness and physician awareness. More patients are being treated early, especially within four months of diagnosis. And doctors now have many new diagnostic and treatment tools, especially new drugs and high-energy radiation, that are effective against cancer. These same factors will save more than one hundred thousand lives this year (1978).

The most commonly chosen parameter to measure survival and indicate curability of cancer is the five-year survival rate. Five-year survival is a good manner of judging cure after cancer of the stomach or rectum. For other cancers, such as tonsil, tongue, and larynx, two-year survival gives a very good estimate of cure. But such lesions as breast cancer and malignant melanoma can recur after five years. Ten-year survival is a better way to judge cure of these tumors.

More women survive cancer than men. In a study by the National Cancer Institute, the cases of 219,493 white and 21,-088 black patients whose cancers were diagnosed between 1955 and 1964 were studied. Significant differences were found. Half of the white women in the study but only a third of the white men survived five years after diagnosis. The reason for this disparity is obscure but probably is related to the fact that in general women live longer and are healthier than men.

Cancer survival is also affected by race. In the same National Cancer Institute study, two-fifths of the black women and less than a fourth of the black men survived five years. This racial disparity puzzles the N.C.I. There is no evidence that blacks in the study received less care than whites. One possible explanation could be that the immune systems of blacks and whites respond differently to cancerous growths. The N.C.I. analysis showed that, even when their cancers were diagnosed at the same stage of development, whites lived longer than blacks, with a few notable exceptions. But black or white, cancer patients can take three important steps to assure themselves the best chance of surviving their disease.

First, know cancer's danger signals. Sudden change in bowel habits, abnormal bleeding, changes in a wart or mole, breast lumps, or hoarseness that persists for more than two weeks should receive a physician's prompt attention.

Second, regular checkups are important. These should include a chest X ray, sigmoidoscopic exam of the rectum, and, for women over forty a breast examination with X-ray mammography, since the slight risks of mammography are greatly outweighed by the potential benefits. A Pap smear of the cervix should be done on all adult women.

Third, if cancer or signs of it are discovered, a large cancer center should be sought out for further diagnostic efforts and treatment. As the great Dr. James Ewing, a pioneer cancer researcher, reported in 1929, "We have been forced to conclude that the treatment of many major forms of cancer can no longer by wisely entrusted to the unattached general physician or surgeon, or to the general hospital as ordinarily equipped, but must be recognized as a specialty requiring special training, equipment, and experience."

Dr. Ewing's observation is truer today than it was in the twenties. The treatment of cancer is a sophisticated medical discipline, one requiring highly trained specialists and elaborate, expensive equipment unlikely to be found in smaller institutions. The alert cancer patient should entrust his or her care to a university hospital connected with a medical school, preferably a hospital specializing in the treatment of cancer.

But above all, keep in mind that too much surgery is being performed in the United States today, and this includes cancer surgery. The prestigious American College of Surgeons itself acknowledges that there is a great oversupply of surgical practitioners. And though half as many operations are done in the United Kingdom, Britons are healthier than Americans on the average.

In the past, surgery was the only means of controlling cancer. Today high-energy radiotherapy has been so perfected that it may produce the same cure rates as surgery in many forms of cancer, without the disfigurement or complications resulting from a surgical procedure. So before considering any form of cancer surgery, a patient should consult a qualified radiation therapist.

2 Breast Cancer

The magnitude of the breast cancer problem is much greater than is generally realized. It is the number one killer of women in the United States. There are roughly seventy thousand new cases each year, with thirty-one thousand deaths.

The enormity of these figures is hard to comprehend unless they are translated into the experiences of our everyday life. The new cases of breast cancer each year would fill Yankee Stadium with standing room only. More women develop breast cancer than the total automobile accident deaths in the United States each year. In ten years, the incidence of breast cancer exceeds the population of Boston. In ten years of the Vietnam War, while the United States lost thirty-seven thousand servicemen in Southeast Asia, three hundred and ten thousand women died from cancer of the breast. One out of every fifteen newborn girls will develop cancer of the breast. In every seventeen-minute period, three new cases of breast cancer will be diagnosed, and in those same seventeen minutes, one woman will die of cancer of the breast. In the U.S. population, the mortality rate of cancer of the breast has remained very nearly twenty-five per hundred thousand women over the past forty years.

Yet in spite of these facts, most women are unaccustomed to examining themselves regularly to find breast masses. And when a woman does find such a mass, she often hesitates to visit a doctor. She fears being told that she has cancer, she fears the treatment, and she fears the consequences of her illness —must she sacrifice her breast?

The breast is actually a large, specialized sweat gland; it is similar to its smaller cousins, the apocrine sweat glands. These are found primarily under the arms and produce the aromatic sweat associated with sexual arousal. The breast tissue begins to develop during the sixth week of intrauterine life. At birth, there are fifteen to twenty primary milk ducts.

Unlike leukemia, which was only identified in the nineteenth century, breast cancer was recognized and feared even by ancient peoples. Egyptian medical papyruses have been found describing breast masses, and medieval manuscripts showing breast tumors and illustrating breast amputation survive to this day.

Until the nineteenth century, however, physicians were unable to treat breast cancer in an effective manner. Crude surgical techniques, the lack of anesthetic agents, and postoperative infections and other complications made the treatment often as horrible as the disease. The discovery of ether, the development of germ-free surgery, and refined surgical techniques combined to lend themselves to the development of the first effective treatment for breast cancer.

William S. Halsted, the greatest American surgeon of the nineteenth century, devised the radical mastectomy in the 1890s. Halsted found that this operation, which removed the affected breast, the muscles beneath, and the lymph nodes under the adjacent arm, offered the best chance of survival. Halsted made many other valuable contributions to surgery: the introduction of rubber gloves during operations and the Halsted repair of hernia are two of his better-known innovations.

But at the time Halsted was refining the radical mastectomy, a European discovery was made that was to affect the treatment of all forms of cancer. In 1896, Wilhelm Roentgen discovered X rays; a few years later, Marie Curie isolated radium. Within a short time, radiation was found to be an effective agent in the treatment of many forms of cancer, so effective, in fact, that today in some types of cancer, either radiation or surgery may be used. One type of cancer that may be amenable to either form of therapy is cancer of the breast.

Recent evidence suggests a rise in both the incidence of breast cancer and its mortality. Several other curious facts have also been proved. Breast cancer is more common in the left breast than in the right; it is twice as common in Jewish women as in non-Jews, and it is 1.5 times as common in single women as in married women. Women without children are more likely to be affected, as are women who have not breast fed. A woman may develop cancer in both breasts in 4 percent or more cases. Men may rarely develop breast cancer; for every hundred female cases, there is one male case. There is also a fivefold increase in the incidence of breast cancer among people whose close relatives have contracted the disease.

The best chance for survival, of course, is in the patient whose cancer is detected early. A cancer will typically present as a lump in the breast, which in the early stages is isolated, moveable, and painless. As the cancer advances, fixation of the lesion, retraction of the skin or nipple, ulceration, pain, redness, and enlarged lymph nodes under the arm may appear; any of these signs suggests a poorer outlook than for the patient with early disease. If the lump in the breast has been present for one month, the cancer will have spread to the lymph nodes under the adjacent arm in 50 percent of cases. If the lump in the breast has been present for six months, the nodes will be involved in 68 percent of cases.

In spite of many years of research, the cause of breast cancer, as of all cancer, remains obscure. Viruslike particles have been found in the milk of women with breast cancer, but similar particles have been found in normal women. Recently, diets low in animal fats have been found to be associated with lower breast cancer incidence; the Japanese fish and rice diet is associated with the lowest incidence of breast cancer of any country studied. Injury to the breast and the use of birth control pills do not appear to cause breast cancer, although certain hormones can influence the course of the disease.

The simplest technique to detect breast cancer is, of course, palpation. This should be done gently and thoroughly with the breast in different positions. Feeling under the arm for lumps—enlarged lymph nodes—is often the manner in which cancer is first discovered; in a large breast, the initial lesion often cannot be felt until very late.

Fourteen years ago the technique of mammography was first introduced. This valuable screening method uses X rays to detect small breast lesions and lesions in large breasts that would otherwise not be palpable. Over 90 percent of the cancers discovered in this way have not spread to other parts of the body.

A recent innovation in mammography, called xeromammography, uses the process of xerography, the duplicating process, instead of X-ray film to record the breast image. The edges of structures in the breast are delineated more sharply by this technique; arteries and veins can also be visualized. But a hot dispute still rages between film mammographers and xeromammographers as to which examination is best. And a third method is also being tried.

The human body radiates heat, and this phenomenon is taken advantage of in thermography. While the heat radiated by the breasts should be relatively uniform, breast lesions are sometimes hotter or colder than the surrounding normal tissues, making their detection possible on thermograms. Critics of thermography maintain, though, that some lesions still go undetected; nonexistent lesions are also frequently identified. For this reason, a thermogram should not be considered a substitute for other techniques.

Many types of noncancerous growths occur within the breast and can be seen on mammograms. Seventy percent of these masses may be merely cystic collections of fluid, fiber, or fat. The breast changes during the menstrual cycle; certain lumps may appear and disappear. Some women with a disorder called fibrocystic disease of the breast have innumerable cystic lesions in both breasts. This disorder is troublesome only because it may mask the development of breast cancer.

Cancer of the breast arises most frequently in the small ducts and ductules that transport milk. The outer, upper fourth of the breast is most frequently affected. From its site of origin, the cancer usually first spreads to the lymph nodes under the adjacent arm; bone is the most common site next involved; brain, liver, and lung may also be affected.

A mammogram can often differentiate a harmless lesion from cancer, but the only definitive diagnostic technique is biopsy. A small piece of tissue is taken from the mass and examined microscopically. If cancer is detected, the mode of treatment employed depends upon whether the cancer has spread.

Distant cancer may be obvious when the patient is first seen by the physician. Cancer in bone may cause severe pain, or it may cause a bone to fracture. A chest X ray will quickly reveal any large deposits of cancer in the lungs. Until recently, however, small bone lesions that did not produce symptoms could not be detected. Small liver and brain lesions were also difficult to locate. Removing the breast of a patient with such lesions is, of course, like closing the stable gate after the horse has run off. But within the last few years, a new medical technique, radioisotope imaging, has been developed that is sensitive enough to find asymptomatic distant cancer.

Certain chemical compounds, when introduced into the body, will localize in specific regions. If these compounds are labeled with a radioactive element, their presence may be detected by the radiation they emit. The compound technetium 99m diphosphonate can be used to visualize the entire skeleton to detect small cancerous bone lesions. Another compound, technetium 99m sulfacolloid, can be used to find liver lesions, and a third compound, technetium 99m pertechnetate, can identify lesions within the brain. The examinations using these compounds—the bone scan, the liver scan, and the brain scan—are now performed on all patients with breast cancer prior to treatment.

Even though bone, liver, and brain may be ostensibly free of cancer, certain "criteria of inoperability" may make the outlook for the breast cancer patient worse. These are swelling of the skin over the breast, lumps in the skin over the breast, lumps in the skin around the ribs or breastbone, swelling of the adjacent arm, tumor present in lymph nodes above the collar bone, or redness and ulceration of the skin of the breast. Most surgeons will not operate if any of these is present; even if all are absent, however, the correct course of action is still the subject of disagreement.

In all of medicine, the treatment of localized cancer of the breast is one of the most hotly disputed and virulently argued topics, and the value of various treatment methods has been challenged again and again. Although radical mastectomy is claimed by some to yield the best survival rate statistically, analysis of results from a variety of treatments shows only moderate variation in overall survival from the least therapy to the most radical mastectomy.

Within the past few years, series of patients have been treated by excision of only the breast lump ("lumpectomy") followed by radiation therapy. This simple and nondisfiguring form of therapy achieved the same survival rates as in patients treated by radical mastectomy in the same hospital.

Another form of treatment is the simple mastectomy, in which only the affected breast is removed; the muscles and lymph nodes are left behind. When this is combined with radiation therapy, the so-called McWhirter technique, the survival results are again comparable with those of other forms of therapy. And these simpler methods have an advantage. They provide fewer problems to the patient.

The radical mastectomy has the highest rate of complications after surgery of all forms of treatment for breast cancer. Besides being cosmetically disfigured, the woman often needs special exercises to regain full use of her arm. One of the most disagreeable and disfiguring complications of radical mastectomy is lymphedema of the arm; in this not uncommon condition, the removal of the lymph nodes under the arm leaves no adequate drainage for fluid in the tissues. The affected arm may swell to enormous proportions, causing pain, disability, and ineffable disfigurement. Worst of all, this distressing condition is lifelong and untreatable when it occurs.

Complications of both simple and radical mastectomies are infections in the surgical wound, which can be persistent, and inadequate healing of the wound with death of tissue; skin grafting may be needed in cases where the wound will not heal. And lifelong disfigurement because of loss of a breast is inevitable. Only after lumpectomy and radiation therapy is there usually no disfigurement.

Radiation therapy has also been employed as the *only* mode of treatment in breast cancer patients. Dr. Leonard R. Prosnitz of the Yale University School of Medicine has recently reported one series of patients who survived as often as those treated by other methods. A similar group of patients treated only with radiation by Dr. Eric Weber of the Harvard Medical School has shown equally encouraging results. Even when surgery is not used on a patient because cancer has spread to the lymph nodes, radiation can still produce cures. In one study, Dr. Ruth Guttman in New York's Delafield Hospital obtained survival rates close to those of the most favorable surgically treated cases.

Yet in spite of these encouraging findings, many surgeons continue to employ the old radical mastectomy. A survey made at the spring, 1975 meeting of the American College of Surgeons demonstrated that the members of this prestigious organization may be paying little attention to reports that question the value of mastectomy in treating breast cancer. Most of the older members said they would still operate even after the cancer had spread to the lymph nodes. But in more advanced disease, neither radiotherapy nor surgery is the whole answer.

There is as yet no means of curing a patient whose breast

cancer has spread to distant sites such as bone, brain, or liver. Some forms of treatment, however, have value in relieving pain or discomfort.

Radiation therapy is one of the mainstays of treatment in advanced breast cancer. Not only is it capable of relieving the pain caused by lesions in bone; it can also promote healing of cancer-filled bones that fracture. Radiation is also of value in controlling symptoms produced by breast cancer that has spread to the brain.

Interference with body hormone production and administration of hormones can relieve symptoms of breast cancer and sometimes temporarily halt growth of lesions. Removal of the ovaries prevents the release of estrogen, the female sex hormone they produce. Removal of the adrenal glands prevents the production of other hormones that can speed the growth of the cancer. Destruction of the pituitary gland is sometimes also performed. The male sex hormone, testosterone, can impede the development of cancer cells and is frequently given to relieve pain.

In the past twenty-five years, many chemical agents have been discovered that are beneficial in the treatment of cancer. Some of these have special value in cancer of the breast. At a recent National Cancer Institute Conference on Breast Cancer in Bethesda, Maryland, attention was focused on the drug L-phenylalanine mustard (L-PAM). Studies showed that patients with underarm lymph node involvement who were given this drug had consistently better results and longer pain relief than those patients receiving no drug. The difference was particularly marked among women under fifty, though the same trend, although less dramatic, was noted among patients over fifty. The National Cancer Institute was so impressed with the results that it has ordered that all women under fifty now being studied be placed on L-PAM.[1]

---

1. Another drug regimen—cytoxan, methotrexate, and 5-Fluorouracil (CMF) —shows even more promise.

Because of better techniques of detection and more public awareness, cases of cancer of the breast are being cured in increasing numbers; this year, 39,000 women will be cured. But the psychological aspects of the disease are also important. While in some cases a mastectomy will bring a husband and wife closer together, in others there will be a divorce. Today, programs such as the American Cancer Society's Reach to Recovery are attempting to deal with problems such as this. These programs help survivors of breast cancer who feel like outcasts communicate with other women who have had a mastectomy and who have overcome their difficulties.

Treatment of breast cancer has come a long way in the past hundred years. I hope some day we will see the end of this number-one killer and crippler of women.

3 Lung Cancer

Cancer of the lung has become the most frequent form of cancer in men in the United States and many other countries. Considered a rarity at the turn of the century, the disease struck sixty-four thousand American men and fifteen thousand American women in 1974. Every year younger and younger individuals are being afflicted.

Cancer of the lung is a lethal disease. When they are first seen, 50 percent of all patients with this tumor cannot be operated on for cure. Of the 50 percent who can have surgery, half will be found to have a growth so extensive that the surgeon cannot remove it all. Only 5 percent of all lung cancer patients will survive five years. Such a fortunate patient was John Wayne. Walt Disney, like most victims, was not so lucky. Why?

Cure of lung cancer, or bronchogenic carcinoma, is infrequent because tumor cells metastasize early. And in the incurable cases, death comes swiftly; from the time of discovery, the average patient will survive six to nine months with only one-fifth living over a year.

The fantastic increase in cancer of the lung has resulted in the most extensive research ever devoted to any disease. Regrettably, all of this effort has resulted in minuscule progress in early detection and treatment methods. Breakthroughs in treatment of other forms of cancer have done little to alter lung cancer's grim survival statistics.

The most well-known factor causative of lung cancer is, of

course, smoking, more particularly the inhaling of tobacco smoke. The complex chemical mixture in tobacco smoke has been found to contain known cancer-producing compounds. Yet between 1920 and 1955, cigarette consumption in the United States increased fourfold for all persons over fourteen years of age and is still increasing today, in spite of the grim warning the law now requires printed on every cigarette pack and cigarette ad.

The connection between lung cancer and smoking is not a loose one. The risk increases with the number of cigarettes smoked per day and the length of the smoking habit. A man who smokes two packages of cigarettes daily has a one-in-ten chance of developing cancer of the lung. If he smokes in excess of two packages per day, this hypothetical man is sixty times more likely to get lung cancer than a man who never smoked. A smoker who coughs is twice as likely to get a lung cancer as a smoker who does not. But if a smoker uses a hookah, as did the wise caterpillar in *Alice's Adventures in Wonderland,* his chances of lung cancer are significantly reduced!

Organic and inorganic industry-related chemicals as causes of cancer of the lung are incriminated in a large amount of evidence. Arsenic used on vines resulted in lung cancer of Beaujolais vine growers until this pesticide was discontinued. Colorado uranium miners have a lung cancer incidence four times what would be expected, indicating that radiation from the uranium ore must have something to do with the production of lung cancer. In addition, asbestos, chromium, nickel, iron, isopropyl oil, coal tar fumes, and petroleum oil mists all have been shown to increase the risk of cancer in those who work with these substances.

Socioeconomic level and air quality influence the development of lung cancer. One study of the residents of New Haven, Connecticut, showed a 40 percent greater incidence among the poor than among other economic classes. In another study, men living in cities were found to be at greater risk than those who lived in the country. Industrial pollution of the air, particularly of large cities, no doubt is responsible for this phenomenon.

The type of cancer cell that forms the tumor greatly affects survival in lung cancer patients. If the lesion is made up of undifferentiated small cells, also called oat cells, the patient almost certainly will not live a year. But if squamous cells, adenocarcinoma, or large cells are involved, chances for cure are somewhat better.

Tumors of the lung often grow more silently than other forms of cancer. Sometimes the first symptoms are produced by tumor that has metastasized to another part of the body. And when symptoms do appear in the lung, they are often not alarming. Even a physician consulted may tend to pass them off.

The earliest symptom of lung cancer is usually an irritating cough, sometimes occurring at night, accompanied by the production of sputum or phlegm. Chest pain, blood-streaked sputum, and shortness of breath also commonly appear. Some patients may be affected by changes in other parts of the body before lung symptoms; these may be classified as follows:

1. hormonal abnormalities
2. nerve and muscle changes, including muscle wasting
3. skin changes, especially darkening of skin under arms and regions of skin inflammation
4. changes in the finger bones and nails, with the tongue-twisting name of hypertrophic pulmonary osteoarthropathy
5. blood vessel inflammation, inflammation of the valves of the heart
6. anemia and blood-clotting abnormalities

When lung cancer is suspected, a chest X ray is the most commonly employed tool to document the disease. The cancer shows up as a white spot against the darker background of the uninvolved lung. But because other diseases unrelated to cancer cause the same X-ray changes, additional steps are generally taken to confirm the diagnosis. It's embarrassing to treat a patient for what seems to be cancer, but later turns out to be tuberculosis.

An easy confirmatory test is sputum cytology. A sample of sputum coughed up from the lungs is spread on a slide, stained, and examined. Often cancer cells can be recognized microscopically; if not, bronchoscopy is undertaken.

Until recently, a bronchoscope was a rigid metal tube passed through the mouth and into the lung. A light at the lower end enabled the physician to view the lung; if the cancer could be seen, he removed a portion of it with a forceps inserted through the tube. More recently, special flexible bronchoscopes, called fiberoptic bronchoscopes, have been developed; these can reach much farther and more easily into the distant recesses of the lung. Tissue is retrieved by means of a small brush fastened to the end of a long wire passed through the bronchoscope. If all efforts to obtain cancer cells with the bronchoscope fail, two other diagnostic maneuvers are commonly employed.

The scalene nodes—small lymph nodes in the tissue behind the clavicles (collarbones)—will be found to contain tumor cells in about a fourth of all lung cancer patients. Just a small incision after a local anesthetic has been administered is adequate to extirpate a node for a scalene node biopsy.

A somewhat trickier method for confirming the presence of lung cancer is mediastinoscopy. This is done with an instrument called a mediastinoscope—it's similar to a bronchoscope— that is introduced into the mediastinum, the region between the lungs and behind the sternum (breastbone). Lymph nodes in the mediastinum will contain cancer cells in 75 percent of cases. And if a node on the opposite side of the mediastinum from the tumor is found to have malignant tissue within it, surgery may be avoided because a physician will know that the cancer has definitely spread.

Unfortunately, mediastinoscopy can be treacherous. At a famous hospital in Baltimore a few years ago, an assistant professor of psychiatry underwent this procedure. The mediastinoscopist attempted to cut out a piece of what he thought was a lymph node, but was actually part of a large artery. The forty-year-old psychiatrist bled to death in less than half a minute.

In 1933, Dr. Evarts A. Graham successfully removed the first cancerous lung. His patient, a physician, survived twenty-nine years without evidence of cancer and outlived Dr. Graham, who succumbed, ironically, to lung cancer. Today, if the cancer is close to the periphery of the lung near the ribs and the chest wall, surgery is considered the best form of treatment. Either a portion of the lung (lobectomy) or the whole lung (pneumonectomy) will be removed, depending on the size of the tumor and what shape the other lung is in.

But surgery should never be performed on lung cancer patients once the cancer has spread; radiation therapy is indicated here. The principal goal of radiation in such cases is palliation, the relief of distress symptoms: cough, coughing up blood, and pain. Good palliation can be expected in 80 percent of cases.

In a small percentage of tumors, radiation therapy may be curative. One study reported that 30 percent of small lung lesions could be completely eradicated with radiation alone. But such small tumors are also the best candidates for surgical removal. With everything considered, surgery is likely to be a better bet.

The type of radiotherapy delivered to lung cancers, as well as to most other types of cancer, is supervoltage radiation. This may be obtained from cobalt sixty or another high-energy source such as a linear accelerator or betatron. During treatment the patient lies under the machine and the X rays are delivered externally.

In the past, radiation of lower energies, called orthovoltage or 250 KEV radiation, was in common use. But the lower energies produced severe and permanent radiation skin reactions. With a few notable exceptions, such as skin cancers, orthovoltage radiation is now considered poor therapy for most conditions.

In recent years, certain anticancer drugs have been tried on lung cancer patients with the hope that their life span might be increased and their quality of life improved. So far, these drugs have never been demonstrated to prolong life. In some cases, though, they may be helpful in relieving symptoms.

The ocean of bad news about lung cancer might seem deep enough to down the greatest optimist, but one drop of hope does exist—better survival through early detection. Lung cancer is present for several months before it is visible on chest X ray; it is seen on chest X ray almost twenty months before symptoms develop. When syptoms appear, patients delay an average of three months before seeking medical advice, and since lung cancer may mimic other diseases, the doctor generally delays another four months to attempt to clear up the patient's symptoms with antibiotics. Thus more than twenty-seven months have elapsed before lung cancer—now probably incurable—is diagnosed. How can this process be speeded up?

Major studies are now under way at Johns Hopkins Hospital and the Mayo Clinic using early detection methods on high-risk patients—males over forty-five years of age with a twenty-year history of smoking more than one pack of cigarettes per day. "Stage zero" cases are found by routine examinations of sputum for malignant cells.

During the last thirty years, thirty patients with stage zero lung cancer have been seen at New York City's Memorial Hospital. In twenty-two, the cancer was promptly located and surgery performed; 60 percent of this group was cured. But in the remaining patients, whose tumor was not promptly found, the dismal cure rates for ordinary cases prevailed.

So the family doctor is the person who holds the key to better survival after lung cancer. He should maintain a high index of suspicion and perform routine chest X rays and sputum tests on high-risk patients. Chest X rays alone are not enough. Obviously, an improved diagnostic technique is urgently needed. A blood test for lung cancer would probably be ideal and is now being sought. But for the present, screening with a chest X ray every six months, perhaps in March and September, combined with a sputum test every six months, in June and December, can detect more cancers at an early stage and result in a significantly higher rate of survival.

4 Cancer of the Female Reproductive Organs

Cervix

Cancer of the cervix is the second-most-common form of cancer in American women, exceeded only by breast cancer. Lurleen Wallace, governor of Alabama and wife of a prominent American politician, was still a young woman when cervical cancer caused her tragic and untimely death. But greater public awareness of this disease is bringing more patients to a physician at an early, curable stage.

The cervix is a cylindrical structure, the "neck" of the uterus, that caps the upper end of the vagina. A small central opening, the external os, leads into the uterus. In a woman who has had no children, the os is small and symmetric. The os of a woman with children is stretched and sometimes chronically infected. This infection increases susceptibility to cervical cancer, and so do other factors.

Cancer of the cervix has an intriguing distribution profile. It is most common among poor women, especially if they happen to be black or Puerto Rican. Among women from any racial or economic group, it occurs most often among those who begin sexual activity as teenagers or have many sexual partners. On the other hand, cervical cancer is extremely rare among nuns. And, perhaps surprisingly, the disease is also seldom seen in Jewish women. One factor that may distinguish Jewish women from others is that they have intercourse mainly or exclusively with circumcised men.

Is there a relationship among the predisposing factors that might suggest a causative agent for cervical cancer? Researchers noted that this distribution profile is similar to that for venereal disease. Suspicion soon centered on a sexually transmitted organism, the herpes simplex type two virus.

The majority of patients with herpes infections—now increasing epidemically because of the new sexual freedom—are teenage girls and unmarried women. Symptoms generally start from three to seven days after exposure. Mild tingling and burning sensations of the genitalia are followed by pustular, whitish lesions on a red base, the familiar "cold sores." There may be only one attack, or repeated flare-ups can be troublesome for years.

Microscopic examination of secretions in patients with cervical cancer reveals cells with small particles within them characteristic of herpesvirus infections. Efforts to isolate viruses from cervical cancer specimens have yielded predominantly herpesvirus type two. And antibody changes also incriminate the virus.

Antibodies are complex proteins within the blood, formed by the body's immune system to protect against invading organisms. The presence of specific antibodies is good presumptive evidence of infection. Controlled, careful studies have shown that significantly more antibodies to herpesvirus type two are found in women with cervical cancer than in normal women. In fact, women with antibodies to herpesvirus type two are ten times more likely to have advanced cervical cancer than women without them, seven times more likely to have cervical cancer, and six times more likely to have severe premalignant cervical changes.

Researchers have theorized that circumcised males are less likely than other men to harbor and transmit the virus—hence the rarity of the disease among Jewish women. There is also evidence that the cervical cells of teenagers, which are still developing, are more vulnerable to virus-induced precancerous changes than are the cervical cells of mature women. This would explain the high incidence of the disease among women who began sexual activity early. Intercourse with many partners would of course increase a woman's chances for contact with a carrier of the virus.

Is there a relationship between other forms of venereal disease and the development of cervical cancer? Apparently not. In one comparison of cervix cancer patients and normals, no significant difference was found in the incidence of trichomonas or syphilis, but the cancer patients did have markedly more herpesvirus type two.

Ninety-five percent of cervical cancer cases are epidermoid cancer, so called because they arise from cells just at the opening of the cervical os. But another five percent of cases are adenocarcinomas that arise within the cervical canal. Adenocarcinoma is unrelated to the herpes virus, to intercourse with many partners, or to the partner's circumcision or lack of it. Nuns and Jewish women are as frequently afflicted as others.

No other form of cancer offers the opportunity of early detection that is presented by cancer of the cervix. One test, the Papanicolaou test or Pap test, can document the presence of the disease in its earliest stage, *carcinoma in situ,* before the cancer cells have broken through a so-called basement membrane that separates them from the remainder of the cervical tissue. In a Pap test, cells taken from the cervix with a wooden spatula are smeared on a slide and examined microscopically for evidence of malignancy.

Carcinoma in situ is almost 100 percent curable. Unfortunately, there usually are no symptoms at this stage. For the symptomatic later stages, cure rates drop off dramatically.

The earliest symptoms that could betray the existence of a small cervical cancer may give no concern: prolongation of the menstrual period, watery discharge, and slight vaginal bleeding between periods. Many women seek medical attention after the most characteristic symptom, bleeding after intercourse. Late signs are yellowish, foul-smelling vaginal discharge and hemorrhage, severe pelvic pain, nausea, vomiting, weight loss, and anemia.

If the Pap test indicates malignancy, a biopsy of the cervix will be performed. This is done with a small tissue punch not too much different in appearance from a one-hole paper punch. In order to locate the most likely spot to punch, an iodine solution is spread over the cervix. Normal cervical tissue will be stained brown because it contains a carbohydrate called glycogen. The regions containing cancer cells remain unstained because of glycogen depletion. It is these unstained areas that are examined. This locating method is called the Schiller test.

To more precisely locate the position of the cervical lesion, fractional dilatation and curettage (D & C) is helpful. After a general anesthetic such as ether has been administered, finger-like dilators are passed through the cervical os to open it sufficiently to insert a sharp, spoonlike curette. Specimens of tissue are scraped by the curette from the lower and upper parts of the cervix and the uterine cavity and examined separately.

Colposcopy is a technique for locating even more precisely an abnormal area on the surface of the cervix. A visual inspection through the vagina is performed with a special microscope that can magnify ten to twenty times. Lesions invisible to the unaided eye can be clearly seen through the colposcope. This sophisticated method of diagnosis has been very popular in Europe, but only in the last few years have American gynecologists begun to show enthusiasm for it.

Once the diagnosis of cervical cancer has been established with certainty, staging of the lesion to estimate its size is important. The stage of the cancer dictates the method of treatment as well as the patient's chances of survival. While under anesthesia, the woman receives the same type of pelvic examination she received in the gynecologist's office, but muscle relaxation due to the anesthetic enables much more to be palpated than could be otherwise. In addition, special X-ray tests— an intravenous pyelogram to see the urinary tract and a barium enema to see the colon—are done to determine whether the tumor has involved the urinary tract or bowel. The interior of the bladder is also inspected with a special instrument called a cystoscope.

Stage zero cervical cancer is another name for the earliest form of the disease, *carcinoma in situ.* As has been mentioned, this stage has the best survival rate, almost 100 percent. The treatment is usually complete removal of the uterus (hysterectomy). The ovaries will also be taken in a woman past menopause. If, however, the patient wants to have children, cure can be obtained by removing a wide cone or cuff of cervical tissue. Careful follow-up after this procedure to detect any recurrent cancer is, of course, mandatory.

A *stage I cervical cancer* is strictly confined to the cervix and does not involve the remainder of the uterus or any other pelvic structure. Ninety percent of women will survive after adequate treatment. In most hospitals today, radiation therapy is used exclusively. This involves external radiation given with cobalt sixty or another high-energy source combined with radioactive radium or cesium applicators that are introduced through the vagina into the cervix and uterus and left in place two to three days, usually on two separate occasions about two weeks apart.

A *stage II cervical cancer* may extend beyond the cervix and involve the uterus, but it has not spread to the wall of the pelvis. The vagina may also be involved as long as its lower third is free of tumor. Seventy percent of women will survive a stage II lesion after adequate therapy, and this therapy is the same as for stage I.

A *stage III cervical cancer* has extended onto the pelvic wall or involves the lower third of the vagina. Thirty-five percent of patients will survive this lesion after treatment. Therapy here is principally with external irradiation, since the large, bulky tumor mass makes an internal application of radioactive sources quite difficult.

A *stage IV cervical cancer* has invaded the bladder or rectum or extended beyond the limits of the pelvis. Survival with a tumor this extensive drops to 14 percent. Therapy is the same as for the stage III lesion.

Cancer of the cervix discovered during pregnancy presents a special treatment problem. If the cancer is a stage zero lesion, the woman is allowed to deliver the baby, and therapy is undertaken afterward. For a more advanced cancer, an abortion is performed up to the twenty-fourth week of pregnancy, followed by curative therapy. When cancer is found after the twenty-fourth week, the baby is removed by cesarean section as soon as it can survive outside the uterus, and a hysterectomy is done at the same time. Alternatively, radiation therapy may be employed in lieu of hysterectomy. But is one method better? For years, there has been a controversy between surgeons and radiotherapists over the best form of therapy for cervical cancer. True, there is no significant difference in the cure rate following surgery or radiation therapy. Nonetheless, radiation is superior to surgery for two reasons: (1) about 20 percent of patients are inoperable when first seen and (2) the complications occurring after radiotherapy are fewer than after surgery.

The most significant complication of surgery is damage to the urinary tract, which may happen in 7 percent of operations performed by even the most skillful surgeon. A ureter—a muscular tube conducting urine from the kidney to the bladder—can be damaged, resulting in loss of a kidney. Or an abnormal connection, a fistula, may be formed between a ureter and the bowel or the abdominal cavity.

Radiation also causes problems. The bladder or rectum are sometimes damaged by the X rays. Radiation can occasionally cause a bone to break, fistulas to form, or damage to other normal tissue. But these complications should affect less than 5 percent of all patients treated.

Uterus

Cancer of the uterus is becoming increasingly common. The advancing average age of the population is bringing ever larger numbers of uterine cancers to physicians. Because this is one of the most treatable and curable of all forms of cancer, early detection and treatment are of paramount importance.

The uterus is a pear-shaped, muscular organ situated in the middle of the female pelvis. Just in front lies the bladder, and just behind, the rectum. The upper and middle portions of the uterus are referred to as the fundus and corpus respectively;

the lowest portion is the cervix. The uterine walls are composed of thick layers of smooth muscle, and the interior is lined by a thin layer of glandular tissue, the endometrium.

Cancer of the endometrium, an adeno (glandular) carcinoma, is the most common form of uterine cancer. This disease occurs in an older age group than cervical cancer—the majority of cases are past menopause; it is very common in Jewish women and women who have had no children—the exact opposite of cervical cancer. High blood pressure, diabetes, obesity, and a late menopause seem to be predisposing factors. In addition, some investigators feel that abnormally high levels of estrogen, a female hormone, may have a causal relationship.

The most common early sign of uterine cancer is a slight vaginal bleeding. For this reason, any abnormal bleeding in the menopausal and especially postmenopausal woman is regarded with great suspicion by gynecologists, and rightly so, since a history of "bloody menopause" is often found in uterine cancer patients. Uterine polyps—small growths attached to the uterine cavity by a stalk—are also associated with increased uterine cancer after menopause. A malodorous watery vaginal discharge is at times present, and it is a very significant sign of the disease.

If a woman ignores the early signs of uterine cancer, the more ominous late signs appear, heralding poorer chances for survival. Persistent and progressive pain, spreading from the low back to the low abdomen, is what brings many patients to their physician. In more advanced tumors, pieces of dead cancer tissue may actually be eliminated through the vagina.

The only really effective way to diagnose early endometrial cancer is a dilatation and curettage (D & C). The scrapings from the uterine lining obtained with the spoonlike curette are examined microscopically. Obtaining cells with only a Pap test spatula will miss many cancer cases. Abnormal uterine bleeding is so common that gynecologists say if they aren't doing D & C's on two or three patients a week, they're not being conscientious enough.

Most often, the D & C after abnormal bleeding will not reveal cancer; instead, the tissue scrapings may indicate a condition called endometrial hyperplasia, which is medicalese for cell overgrowth. Cystic glandular hyperplasia, the "swiss cheese" endometrium—so called because of the many cystic holes seen within it—is a common cause of benign abnormal bleeding and is probably related to hormonal imbalances. Adenomatous hyperplasia, a glandular overgrowth, is a more dangerous condition, felt by some gynecologists to be precancerous.

No elaborate examinations are used for staging uterine cancer, since the disease is localized to the uterus until very late. One ominous sign during the pelvic examination is an enlarged, boggy uterus. The worst possible finding is deposits of cancer tissue in the vagina; such a patient will rarely survive five years. For earlier cases, the outlook is much better. Why?

The uterus can be considered a sturdy muscular bottle. Its thick walls are a barrier to early cancer spread. It can withstand enormous doses of radiation, doses that would cook any other body organ three times over. So survival after early treated cases of uterine cancer is very good, usually 90 percent or more.

But if the muscular wall of the uterus is invaded by tumor, the survival rate drops to 70 percent. And if the tumor extends to the cervix, only 50 percent of patients will be cured. As in all forms of cancer, prompt, early treatment is essential.

Cure of uterine cancer can be achieved after either surgery or radiation therapy. Elderly, debilitated, or otherwise inoperable patients may receive radiation therapy alone. At present, though, the most desirable therapeutic approach consists of preoperative irradiation followed by surgery.

For a surgical cure to be achieved, total abdominal hysterectomy is best performed, along with bilateral salpingo-oophorectomy. In other words, the uterus, the ovaries, and both Fallopian tubes are removed. In the past, some surgeons removed the pelvic lymph nodes as well, but there is no evidence that doing so increases the overall survival rate.

Preoperative radiation therapy may be given in two ways.

The radiation may be internally administered by means of small radioactive applicators called Heyman capsules. These are introduced through the vagina into the uterus and left in place three days. Or the patient may receive external irradiation with cobalt sixty. Studies have shown, however, that internal irradiation is best, since this method delivers the highest radiation dose to the tumor.

The complications after treatment with radiation and surgery for cancer of the uterus are similar to those for treatment of cervical cancer. Such complications should only occur in a small percentage of cases when the treatment is performed by experienced hands. Damage to the urinary tract with loss of a kidney, hernia occurring in the surgical scar, and abnormal connections called fistulas developing between the vagina and bladder or bowel—these are the rare aftereffects of surgery. The bowel, vagina, or bladder may suffer some damage in less than 5 percent of women receiving radiation.

When uterine cancer is inoperable, treatment with a special drug, the hormone progesterone, is helpful. Progesterone is normally secreted in small quantities by the ovaries during part of the menstrual cycle. The effect is to prepare the uterine lining for implantation of the fertilized egg and raise the body temperature.

We don't know why progesterone is so valuable in treating uterine cancer, especially in women under forty. Many studies have shown tremendous shrinkage of tumor deposits after the administration of high doses of this drug. For example, in advanced cases of uterine cancer, the abnormal cells may metastasize to the lung. Chest X rays made during therapy demonstrate that large lung deposits of such cancer melt away like snow on a spring day. Patients who had been critically ill report a decrease in pain and an increase in the sense of well-being.

Progesterone therapy is not without its hazards, though. If a woman has heart disease, this agent may make the condition worse. And the body is also stimulated to retain water, placing an even greater load on the heart. The gynecologist must carefully follow the condition of the heart and lungs of all women on progesterone therapy.

One type of uterine cancer, the uterine sarcoma, does not obey any of the rules for endometrial cancer. Sarcomas develop from the muscle of the uterus rather than from the lining. Few women with this tumor will live more than two years, in spite of treatment. Fortunately, sarcoma of the uterus is very rare.

Cancer of the Ovary

The two ovaries are situated on either side of the pelvis. They are egglike in shape, and they produce the female hormones estrogen and progesterone, as well as the ova that grow into human beings.

The onset of ovarian cancer is insidious, and symptoms occur late. Despite the advances in surgery and radiotherapy, only 30 percent of women manage to survive. The third most common female malignancy, ovarian carcinoma results in the largest number of deaths.

The incidence of ovarian cancer rises with age. Ten cases per hundred thousand are reported yearly for women thirty-five to thirty-eight years of age; between the ages of sixty-five and sixty-nine, fifty women per hundred thousand are affected. And strangely, the general frequency of this tumor is rising. Surveys in both New York and Connecticut reveal a 15 percent increase in cases from the late 1940s to the early 1960s. The reason for this is unknown.

Because the structure of the ovary is extremely complex, it has the capability of producing a whole range of tumors, benign and malignant, from the simplest cyst to the weird and remarkable dermoid, which often contains teeth. Pathologists who have spent their lives studying ovarian tumors are continually surprised and confounded by the enormous variety of these growths. The symptoms produced, though, are fairly standard.

Two basic types of ovarian cancers, cystic and noncystic, cause two types of symptoms. Women with cystic ovarian cancer have initial symptoms primarily localized to the pelvis: pain, pressure, and pelvic distress caused by the enlarging mass. In the noncystic, solid ovarian cancers, pressure symptoms from a mass are minimal. Instead, the spread of the tumor throughout the abdominal structures leads to digestive symptoms: bloating, cramps, nausea, and severe constipation.

Certain less common solid ovarian tumors are first noticed because of the abnormal amounts of hormones they produce. The granulosa-theca cell tumors make excessive amounts of estrogen. In an adult woman, this hormone excess leads to proliferation of the uterine lining, abnormal uterine bleeding, and menstrual irregularities. Granulosa-theca cell tumors in a young girl cause precocious puberty. A six-year-old girl so afflicted will be fully sexually developed. The arrhenoblastoma, also called a sertoli-leydig cell tumor, manufactures excessive amounts of testosterone, the male hormone, and causes growth of a beard, clitoral enlargement, male pattern baldness, and greatly increased sexual desire.

Early detection is difficult in ovarian cancer. There is no Pap test or other screening method. Only the skillful hands of a gynecologist performing a pelvic examination can find this growth soon enough to cure it. So visits to her doctor and pelvic examinations twice a year are a must for every adult woman.

And what if the gynecologist does discover a lump or mass in an ovary? Unfortunately, opening the abdomen surgically and removing tissue for microscopic study is the only completely satisfactory way of positively making a diagnosis in early cases. Ovarian cancer is gynecology's great masquerader, and even experienced physicians may mistake it for other conditions. All suspicious pelvic and ovarian masses must be removed for examination; life may depend on it.

Except for obviously far-advanced cases, surgery is the primary form of treatment for ovarian cancer. The uterus, both ovaries, and the Fallopian tubes are taken to remove as much tumor as possible. Sometimes tumors initially too large to re-

move can be reduced to a manageable size after radiation
therapy and drug treatment; therefore, many authorities advise
a "second look" operation after these procedures.
Radiotherapy is administered to ovarian cancer with a high-
energy external source such as cobalt sixty. The abdomen and
pelvis are marked off in strips, and location of the kidneys is
outlined on the skin so that they may be shielded from radiation injury. Each day different strips are irradiated. In the past,
radioactive gold solutions were injected into the abdominal
cavity; this treatment has now been abandoned because of its
poor results.
Today, drug therapy is also playing a role in the treatment
of ovarian cancer. Agents most often used include Cytoxan,
Chlorambucil, Phenylalanine Mustard, and 5-Fluorouracil. Combinations of these compounds produce the best results. Sometimes the response is almost miraculous, and a few women
may even be cured. In some cases, an accumulation of fluid
in the abdominal cavity, called ascites, causes distention and
great discomfort. Radioactive gold is of little value in ameliorating this condition, but drugs give great relief when injected
into the abdomen.
Our best hope for the present in ovarian cancer is in provid-
ing more regular pelvic examinations for all women. But because of the insidious nature of the disease, even this procedure
will probably not find many cancers before they have spread
beyond the ovary and become incurable. Perhaps some day a
reliable screening test to detect early lesions will be developed.
Surgery and radiotherapy will probably offer little more in the
future than they do today. Our best chance appears to be drug
therapy. Maybe before long, we will have a drug that can
effectively alter the course of ovarian cancer.

Cancer of the Vulva and Vagina and Choriocarcinoma
Vulva

The vulva is the outermost part of the female reproductive
tract. The clitoris, the labia majora and minora, and certain
glands are the vulva's component parts.

Carcinoma of the vulva is an uncommon female malignancy, accounting for only 4 percent of genital cancer. Women most frequently affected are between fifty and seventy years old, but the disease seems to appear at an earlier age in black women. A high proportion of patients note a previous dryness and shrinking of the vulva beginning after menopause.

Most vulvar cancers are squamous or skin carcinomas arising from the labia, or lips. Although squamous skin cancers in general have a high cure rate, such cancers of the vulva are an exception. The rich blood and lymphatic supply is often responsible for early spread of the tumor. A small vulvar cancer (less than three centimeters across) can be cured in 70 percent of cases; only 10 percent of patients will live five years after a larger tumor has been treated.

Most cases of cancer of the vulva are preceded or accompanied by itching, worst at night, which may have been present for several years before the appearance of the tumor. Some patients have had a whitish premalignant area called leukoplakia, while others have been diabetic or infected with venereal disease. Usually a palpable lump or nodular area is present, and infection may have occurred as well.

Diagnosis of these lesions is confirmed by removing a piece of tissue for microscopic examination. There is a pitfall, though: two kinds of benign vulvar lesion—with the melodious names of granular cell myoblastoma and syringocystadenoma papilleferum—can easily be mistaken by an inexperienced examiner for cancer. How criminal to remove the vulva of a twenty-five-year-old woman for what turns out to be a simple infection that could have been cured with antibiotics. So a wise patient will have the microscopic slides of a vulvar lesion reviewed by an expert gynecologic pathologist before she allows any therapy to be undertaken.

Radical surgery is the only adequate treatment for vulvar cancer. The entire vulva must be removed (radical vulvectomy) and the adjacent lymph nodes dissected out. Partial removal tried on elderly patients has only yielded disastrous results. After a radical vulvectomy, the surgical defect may heal with surprising rapidity; if not, the open area can be successfully closed with skin grafts. Radiation therapy is of no value in vulvar cancer, except to palliate cases too advanced for surgery.

Vagina

The vagina, or birth canal, is a muscular, membranous, very elastic tube that extends from the vulva to the uterus. Cancer of the vagina is rare, being even less common than cancer of the vulva. The average patient is in her mid-fifties. Black women and Jewish women are rarely afflicted. And one drug has been found to be a causative factor.

In the 1940s and 1950s, the synthetic estrogen compound diethylstilbestrol was given to pregnant women who showed signs of miscarriage. The children of these mothers have been developing a rare form of vaginal cancer, adenocarcinoma of the vagina, in abnormally large numbers. Regular checkups, even during the teenage period, are essential for any girl exposed to diethylstilbestrol *in utero*.

A woman with a vaginal carcinoma usually first notices vaginal discharge, spotting, pain, and groin lumps. Examination of the vagina will reveal the presence of a visible and palpable mass, from which a piece of tissue is taken and examined microscopically to confirm the diagnosis. Chances for survival are best when the lesion is in the upper third of the vagina on the posterior wall.

Radiation therapy can be given for vaginal cancer. Internal radioactive applicators and an external source such as cobalt sixty are used. Recently, radical surgical removal of the entire vagina, uterus, and pelvic lymph nodes has also been employed with some success. Approximately one-third of women with adequately treated vaginal cancer will survive five years.

Choriocarcinoma

Choriocarcinoma of the uterus is a tumor that occurs during pregnancy. Rarely seen in the United States, this disease affects Orientals in disproportionately large numbers.

Choriocarcinoma may develop from a strange growth arising from the placenta, the linking structure between the uterine wall and the umbilical cord. This growth, called a hydatidiform mole, is composed of cysts that grow from the placenta. Such moles are often first identified by the cysts spontaneously eliminated through the vagina and by the abnormal uterine enlargement they cause.

Usually, gynecologists have no difficulty telling the difference between a mole and choriocarcinoma. Chorionic gonadotropin, a protein hormone made by the placenta and used to diagnose pregnancy, is produced in abnormally large quantities by choriocarcinoma. If a hydatidiform mole has been removed and the chorionic gonadotropin levels measured in the blood continue to rise, then the carcinoma is present and treatment is instituted.

Therapy for choriocarcinoma is one of the great success stories of modern medicine. Surgery and radiation therapy had been tried with little success. In 1961, Dr. R. Hertz reported the excellent response of this tumor to the drug methotrexate. Even when distant metastases are present in the lungs and other organs, methotrexate therapy is able to effect amazing cures. Today 70 percent of women survive this once uniformly fatal disease with methotrexate therapy alone.

5 Cancer of the Digestive Tract

Esophagus

The esophagus is a muscular tube, about ten inches long, that transmits food from the mouth to the stomach. A layer of squamous cells—the same type of cell that makes up the skin—lines the interior. From these squamous cells the majority of esophageal cancers arise.

Esophageal cancer commonly affects men over the age of sixty. The disease is most prevalent in Japan, where there are three and a half times as many cases as in the United States. For reasons that are unclear, the incidence is especially high among black men in coastal South Carolina. While males are affected three times more commonly than women in the United States, 40 to 50 percent of Swedish and Finnish patients are women.

As in all forms of cancer, the cause or causes of cancer of the esophagus are unknown. Patients tend to have been heavy smokers and drinkers for many years, as was one famous victim, Ed Sullivan, who was a heavy smoker. Individuals with no teeth or poor teeth seem to be vulnerable, perhaps because the incompletely chewed food traumatizes the lining cells. A particular form of malnutrition in impoverished English, Scotch, and Swedish women, called the Plummer-Vinson syndrome, was long associated with esophageal cancer; addition of iron and vitamins to baking flour has now almost eradicated this condition.

Little distress is generally caused by the earliest manifestation of cancer of the esophagus: a sense of fullness or burning under the sternum (breastbone). The most characteristic symptom is difficulty swallowing—doctors call this "dysphagia"—that the patient can localize precisely to the upper, middle, or lower third of the esophagus. Only one condition, the psychologically induced "globus hystericus," can mimic the swallowing problems. The "globus hystericus" is a psychosomatic symptom generally affecting young or middle-aged women. Such patients complain vigorously about the sensation of a lump in the throat, especially during moments of stress. The presence of a cancer here can easily be ruled out by an X-ray examination. In a real esophageal tumor, the trouble swallowing will continue to get worse. First solid foods must be abandoned, then soft foods; finally, even liquids are swallowed with difficulty. A rapid weight loss inevitably follows the eating problems. And with the advance of the disease come even more ominous signs.

As the cancer becomes larger, it can spread into one of the nerves that activate the vocal cords, the recurrent laryngeal nerve. When this happens, hoarseness will appear. If the tumor spreads into the trachea (windpipe), just adjacent to the esophagus, a persistent cough will trouble the patient, especially when swallowed food passes into the lungs. The worst possible sign is the coughing up of blood, indicating involvement of a large artery; death supervenes within hours after the blood is first seen.

No simple early detection methods exist for esophageal cancer and the initial diagnosis is made by X ray. The patient is given barium sulfate to drink; this liquid is then observed with a fluoroscope as it passes through the esophagus. The ordinarily smooth esophageal walls will be made ragged and irregular by tumor.

If any abnormality is seen on X ray, a positive diagnosis must be made by biopsy and microscopic examination of the tissue obtained. How does a doctor get a piece of tumor from the lower esophagus? A long tube called an esophagoscope is passed through the mouth, and tissue is removed through it with a special forceps. This may sound difficult to accomplish, but circus sword swallowers do the same thing every day of their working lives—without the tissue removal, of course.

Few cases of esophageal cancer are ever cured—probably fewer, in fact, than one in twenty. Many patients, however, can be given great symptomatic relief with proper treatment, especially if the tumor is small and is located in the lower esophagus. Surgical treatment consists of removal of the whole tumor. If the lesion is located close to the stomach, only the cancerous tissue need be removed; the stomach can then be reconnected to the uninvolved esophagus. But if the tumor is in the middle of the esophagus, the entire esophagus must be removed (esophagectomy). To provide a means of swallowing, the surgeon brings up a length of colon and uses the segment to restore continuity to the system, like replacing a bad piece of pipe with a good one.

Unfortunately, surgery has many complications, and some patients will even die on the operating table. Others with but a limited life span spend a considerable time recovering from the operation. Surgeons have tried to improve this situation with a procedure that only requires passing a plastic tube through the tumor. But often radiation therapy can produce comparable cure rates and symptomatic relief without even hospitalizing the patient, allowing him to spend what time he has left at home.

Radiation is given with cobalt sixty or another external high-energy radiation source. The central and symmetric position of the esophagus within the chest allows for treatment in a special manner: the radiation source is rotated around the chest through a complete circle, effectively delivering most of the radiation to the tumor and avoiding damage to normal tissue. The treatments are generally given five days a week for about six weeks. Twenty-five percent of patients will be completely relieved of symptoms, and another 50 percent will experience considerable relief.

Proof of the superiority of radiation to surgery comes from the Edinburgh study of 1,335 patients with esophageal cancer. From 1948 to 1955, the curative treatment was surgery exclusively; from 1956 to 1965, it was surgery for lesions in the lower esophagus and radiation for higher lesions; from 1966 until 1968, high-energy radiation was employed almost exclusively. The better long-term and short-term survival of the irradiated patients was the reason X rays were used instead of surgery in the later years.

Stomach Cancer

Of all the organs of the human body, the stomach is one of the most vulnerable and catered to. Anger leads to burning, and overeating to "acid indigestion," whatever that may be. The advertising profession patronizes the stomach with tablets that absorb forty-seven times their weight in excess acid, powders that fizz, and liquids that coat with an aesthetic pink. Yet despite the impression conveyed by Madison Avenue that the stomach is becoming more delicate in each succeeding generation, susceptibility to one condition has droped precipitously.

Cancer of the stomach is on the decline. According to American Cancer Society figures, only one-fourth as many Americans are afflicted today as in 1930. The United States now has the lowest incidence of any industrial country, although the reason behind this remarkable decrease remains obscure and cannot be attributed to preventive measures.

On the high end of the stomach cancer scale sit Japan, Iceland, and Finland. The basis for the large incidence in these countries remains as mysterious as that for the small number of cases here. The Japanese eat large quantities of smoked fish, and investigators feel that this may have some bearing on the disease. Other researchers believe that a diet high in starch and low in fresh fruits and vegetables ultimately brings on stomach cancer.

More men than women get stomach cancer; the ratio is about

two to one. The disease most often strikes in midlife or later, with peak incidence in the fifty- to fifty-nine-year age group. One recent victim was the great comedian Jack Benny.

Some nonmalignant conditions are predisposing. Small benign tumors—gastric polyps—that grow on a stalk within the stomach may become cancerous. In years past, stomach ulcers were believed to be premalignant; we now know that this is not the case. But one disease is closely associated with stomach cancer: pernicious anemia.

Pernicious anemia is a special form of blood disorder caused by an inability to absorb vitamin B_{12}. Usually this is due to a stomach abnormality. Normal stomachs secrete a protein called intrinsic factor, which is vital for B_{12} absorption; stomachs of pernicious anemia victims do not. In addition, patients with pernicious anemia do not make stomach acid, a condition called achlorhydria by doctors. Fifty years ago, these people didn't live long enough to develop other problems. But a brilliant discovery changed all that.

George Whipple, George Minot, and William Murphy, working on pernicious anemia in the 1920s, won the Nobel Prize in medicine for discovering that the disease could be successfully treated with liver extract, later found to be effective because it contained vitamin B_{12}. When pernicious anemia patients began living longer, 10 percent of them went on to develop stomach cancer. We still don't know the precise reason for this. Undoubtedly, though, the wasting and flattening of the stomach lining that is seen in pernicious anemia is related in some way.

Cancer of the stomach is a silent disease. Symptoms are not usually noticed until the very late, incurable stages. Patients most often complain of vague abdominal discomfort which is not helped by nostrums purchased at the corner drug store. Actual burning, ulcer-type pain is uncommon, but when present generally is not relieved by antacids. Loss of appetite and loss of weight frequently accompany the stomach symptoms, as does the weakness and pallor characteristic of anemia.

Because of misleading and injurious television advertising that promises cures for iron deficiency anemia, or "tired blood," many people do not regard this significant condition with sufficient alarm. The body hoards its iron supply like a miser, and only a menstruating woman is likely to have anemia without other disease. Anemia in a man of any age or in a nonmenstruating woman must be thoroughly investigated, since a serious illness may well be the cause. Taking over-the-counter iron preparations only serves to mask the anemia while delaying proper diagnosis and treatment of the underlying condition.

Certain diagnostic maneuvers are mandatory if symptoms of stomach cancer appear. Stool samples should be tested for the presence of small amounts of blood if anemia is present. Analysis of the stomach secretions for acid should be performed on all stomach ulcer patients. The absence of acid suggests cancer and requires further study if the patient's condition permits.

The X-ray test called an upper gastrointestinal (GI) series is a very accurate method of identifying stomach lesions. Liquid barium sulfate is swallowed by the subject, allowing the stomach and small bowel to be clearly visualized. Skilled interpretation of the resulting X-ray films can usually, but not always, differentiate a benign ulcer from a cancer. The Japanese are especially sophisticated in their X-ray studies on account of their alertness to stomach cancer. Many more early cancers are found and cured in Japan than in the United States.

In recent years, diagnosis of stomach diseases has been improved by the flexible gastroscope. This device may be easily passed into the stomach to allow observation and photography of many different lesions. In addition, a hollow channel in the gastroscope allows special instruments to be passed through in order to obtain tissue specimens of areas in question. Unfortunately, the technique can usually remove only very superficial tissue, which is frequently inadequate for definitive diagnosis.

There are three main types of stomach cancer. The common variety is adenocarcinoma, composed of malignant cells derived from the glands within the stomach. A more uncommon sort of stomach tumor is a lymphoma, derived from lymphoid cells that play a role in immunity. The rarest form is a leiomeiosarcoma, made of malignant cells from the smooth muscle comprising the stomach wall.

Surgery is the best method for treating stomach cancer, but it still leaves much to be desired. The operation most frequently employed is called a Billroth II, named after Dr. Theodore Billroth, the Viennese surgeon who devised the procedure in the late nineteenth century. Most of the stomach is removed from the body during Dr. Billroth's operation. Larger cancers may necessitate removal of the entire organ. And life without a stomach is not exactly pleasant at first.

After a Billroth II, patients have a decreased capacity for food, and frequent small meals are required. A most distressing sequela is the so-called dumping syndrome, in which the remaining stomach empties rapidly, causing intense nausea, sweating, faintness, and weakness. Dumping may follow any meal but is especially likely after foods rich in sugar when taken with fluid. Ninety percent of cases of dumping syndrome will subside spontaneously six months to a year after surgery.

The value of radiation therapy in the treatment of early or potentially curable stomach cancer is unknown. No effort has been made to see whether high-energy X rays would be of value, at least in the United States. In Germany, Dr. R. Sauerbrey irradiated a series of surgically incurable patients and found good relief from symptoms after this treatment. Perhaps in the future, radiation may be found to give better overall results in this disease than surgery.

And the surgical results are dismal. A typical large study done in South Carolina in 1955 revealed the following: Of one hundred patients with stomach cancer, forty-two patients were inoperable, thirty-eight had tumors incompletely removed at surgery, three died as a consequence of surgery, nine died from metastases, leaving eight patients surviving five years.

Bowel Cancer

Small Bowel

In spite of the fact that most of the intestine is made up of small bowel, cancer of the small bowel is rare, less than six cases per million population each year. The reasons for this remarkable invulnerability are obscure. A typical lesion is the strange tumor called a carcinoid. Carcinoid cells manufacture a compound called serotonin, which produces symptoms when the tumor spreads from bowel to liver. These symptoms include intermittent watery diarrhea, abdominal cramps, asthmatic attacks, and heart symptoms caused by damage to valves. Other small-bowel cancers produce bleeding or bowel obstruction. All malignant tumors of the small bowel have a poor outlook: fewer than 20 percent of patients will survive five years.

Large Bowel

The large bowel, or colon, forms the terminal portion of the digestive tract. Undigested residue passes from the small bowel into the colon, where dehydration and elimination occur. Unlike the small bowel, the colon develops cancer with distressing frequency. In the United States in 1970, there were 45,800 deaths from cancer of the colon or its final segment, the rectum. This may be compared with 750 deaths from small bowel cancer, 15,600 deaths from stomach cancer, and 6,100 deaths from esophageal cancer. Yet while colon cancer is the most frequent digestive tract tumor here, it is not so elsewhere.

Finland and Japan have a low incidence of large bowel cancer, and the disease is practically unknown in many South African populations, especially the Bantu. Diet probably plays a large role in the observed disparity. Many researchers suggest that food low in animal fat and refined carbohydrates while high in bulk protects the colon from cancer. True, the Bantu do consume a great deal of animal fat, but they have a very bulky diet. Bantus are frequent defecators, so presumably cancer-inducing materials are in contact with their colon for only a short period of time.

There is no sex difference in the incidence of colon cancer; men and women are equally affected. The disease is one of older patients, with two-thirds being over the age of fifty. Two disorders, however, are associated with the appearance of colon cancer at an earlier age: familial polyposis of the colon and ulcerative colitis.

Familial polyposis of the colon is an inherited condition in which grapelike formations called polyps grow in great quantities from the glandular lining cells. The pattern of inheritance is called Mendelian dominance: if your father or mother had it, there is a 50 percent chance you will too. If the condition is discovered, doctors usually advise total removal of the colon because the chances of developing cancer are so high.

Sometimes a single polyp or two will be found growing in the colon. In the past, doctors suspected that these lesions tended to become cancerous and so removed them prophylactically. Recent statistical studies, though, seem to indicate that there is no more likelihood of cancer developing in a benign polyp than in normal colonic tissue. But one growth, the villous adenoma, does tend to become malignant and should be removed whenever discovered.

Ulcerative colitis is an inflammatory disease of the colon. For reasons unknown, numerous ulcers appear throughout the interior lining. Unlike familial polyposis, it presents severe and immediate symptoms. The unremitting diarrhea and bleeding can usually be controlled with drugs, but after ten years or more, chronic changes in the colon become cancerous in 10 percent of patients.

The distribution of cancer sites within the colon is quite unusual. Twenty-five percent of all cancers begin in the lower portion of the rectum and can be palpated by a doctor's examining finger. Another 50 percent of lesions are within about a foot of this point, easily detectable with the sigmoidoscope, which is a long, lighted tube that can be inserted into the anus. No one knows the reason for this peculiar distribution pattern. Symptoms produced by a colon cancer depend on where the lesion is located. Tumors in the right side of the colon—that portion nearest the connection with small bowel and furthest from the anus—characteristically cause anemia. Tumors in the left side of the colon—the part nearest the anus—lead to bleeding, blood in the stool, and constipation. Rectal tumors give a sensation of incomplete evacuation after a bowel movement. Diarrhea and lower abdominal pain are also frequently encountered complaints. But not uncommonly a far-advanced cancer produces few symptoms or none at all. So early detection would seem imperative. One method, rectal self-examination, will be described at the end of this section.

Another method, sigmoidoscopy, is more difficult to apply. In spite of the sigmoidoscope's ability to find 75 percent of early lesions, the technique is cumbersome and tedious. Four thousand normal patients would have to be examined before one cancer was found. A few years ago there was great hope for the assay of an abnormal blood protein, carcinoembryonic antigen, or CEA, as an easy screening method. But results have been quite disappointing, since CEA appears in the blood in many other conditions besides colon cancer, and it does not even materialize in all cases of colon cancer.

Positive diagnosis of most colon lesions can be made by means of a special X-ray examination, the barium enema. Liquid barium is introduced into the colon and X-ray films are taken. A so-called double contrast enema requires the instillation of air after the barium has been evacuated; this procedure is most helpful in finding polyps and smaller lesions.

Recently, a new instrument, the colonoscope, has come into use. This is a special long tube composed of optical glass fiber bundles that can be passed into the colon and allow visualization of the whole interior surface from the anus to the connection with the small bowel. In addition, a small channel in the colonoscope permits polyps to be removed and biopsy tissue specimens to be taken with a special forceps from any region desired. Once a definitive diagnosis has been made, treatment can begin.

In past years, tumors of the colon and rectum were treated by an approach that was strictly surgical, as this form of cancer was erroneously believed to be insensitive to radiation. If the tumor was above the rectum, a complete removal could be made and the two cut ends of bowel reconnected, a method referred to as anterior resection. But with the rectum involved, a technique called abdominoperineal resection or the Miles operation has been traditionally used. First devised in 1908, the Miles operation is the procedure dreaded by cancer sufferers because it results in loss of the rectum, a colostomy, and impotence in men.

And the survival of patients after surgical treatment of cancer of the rectum or the short, S-shaped segment just above it, the sigmoid, is dismal. For the past twenty years, only one out of every three patients treated with surgery alone has survived five years. Various anticancer drugs have been tried without success. But recently, new approaches have cast a fresh light on therapy.

Numerous investigators have now tried preoperative radiation therapy in cancers of the rectum and sigmoid and have found it to be undeniably effective in increasing survival. Those using this method include Dr. Bernard Roswit and hospitals of the Veterans Administration, Dr. W. Rider at the Princess Margaret Hospital in Toronto, and Dr. S. Raffla at the Brooklyn Methodist Hospital. Of course, preoperative radiation cannot save the rectum, but bigger, curative doses of radiation can; an early case in point was that of William Powell.

> A whole generation has grown up since William Powell was a matinee idol noted for his sophisticated suavity in *The Thin Man, The Great Ziegfield,* and *My Man Godfrey.* . . . But less inevitable than his fading reputation was the actor's actual survival [intact after rectal cancer]. . . .
>
> "I began bleeding from the rectum in March of 1935," he said. "The doctor found a cancer smaller than the nail of your little finger between three and four inches up in-

side my rectum. They recommended removal of the rectum. Then I'd have had to have a colostomy and evacuate into a pouch through an artificial opening for the rest of my life. I didn't feel I could go for this. But the doctors said that for my particular case they could offer an alternative: a temporary colostomy and radiation treatment. I took it."

Surgeons made an incision in Powell's abdomen, brought out part of the colon, and cut it halfway through. "From then on," said Powell, "fecal matter went no farther than this opening in my abdomen and emptied into a pouch attached around my middle."

With the lower colon inactivated, surgeons removed the cancer. Apparently it had not spread. As a further precaution, radiologist Orville Meland of the Los Angeles Tumor Institute implanted platinum needles containing tiny radium pellets.

"For the next six months we simply waited," Powell recalls. "I had a lot of examinations but led a reasonably normal life. I did quite a few radio shows, though I couldn't make movies. The worst thing about the situation was the esthetics of it."

After six months with the cancer apparently eradicated, the surgeons hooked up Powell's intestines the way nature had arranged them originally, after which he continued to have normal body functions. As late as 1955, he played in *Mr. Roberts.* Says Powell simply, "I was one of the lucky ones."[1]

For nearly half a century, there have been scattered reports on cases such as William Powell's indicating that local removal of a rectal tumor is as effective as the Miles operation and colostomy. The first large-scale study was reported by Dr. George Crile, Jr., of the Cleveland Clinic, in 1972. Dr. Crile found that local removal of the tumor was, indeed, as good as

---

1. Reprinted by permission from *Time,* The Weekly Newsmagazine; Copyright Time, Inc. 1963.

the Miles operation. And if the procedure should fail, the rectum could always be removed subsequently. Dr. John Madden, at New York's St. Clare's Hospital, has achieved similar results. Another method of local treatment was reported by Dr. Jean Papillon at the Centre Leon-Berard in Lyon, France. Dr. Papillon inserted a high output X-ray tube through the rectum to give large doses of radiation to the rectal tumor itself and achieved better results than those from the Miles operation. Dr. Ben Sischy of the Highland Hospital in Rochester, N.Y. is now employing Papillon's method with great success.

What do these approaches mean to the colon cancer patient? If the tumor can be removed by an anterior resection with restoration of normal bowel function, all well and good. But if a Miles operation with colostomy is recommended, perhaps the consumer should consider seriously the more conservative methods mentioned. You may not be William Powell. You may not have your style in love scenes with Myrna Loy cramped by a colostomy. But a rectum is still a nice thing to have.

Rectal Self-Examination

But how can rectal tumors be detected early enough so that the conservative methods of treatment can be successfully used? There is one simple, easy-to-apply method—rectal self-examination.

Rectal self-examination is performed most aesthetically during a shower. The arm is extended around the back, rather than through the legs, and the middle finger is inserted gently into the rectum, palm upward. Commercially available lubricants such as KY Lubricating Jelly or Vaseline may be applied to the finger. Alternately, a mild soap such as Ivory may also be used, though some people may find this too irritating. With a little practice, the entire circumference of the lower rectal wall may be palpated. Men, in addition, should be able to feel the prostate gland as a large elevation at the front of the rectum.

If the public can be taught to accept and practice rectal self-

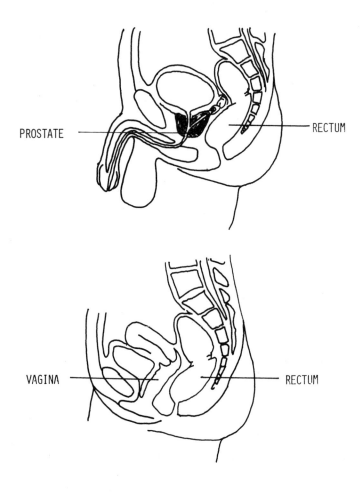

PROSTATE —————————— RECTUM

VAGINA ——————— RECTUM

Rectal Self-Examination
The rectal wall should feel smooth and moist to the touch. Any irregular, hardened areas or warty growths should be reported to a physician. The prostate should be felt to have a firm, regular texture. Any hardened areas, nodules, or swellings in the prostate should be examined by a urologist, as these may be a sign of prostate cancer.

examination regularly, most of the 25 percent of colon cancers within reach of the finger will be detected early enough for a high chance at cure without colostomy. In the year 1978, for example, this figure could approach twenty-five thousand cases in the United States alone.

Pancreatic Cancer

Pancreatic cancer is a relatively rare disease, accounting for not more than 3 percent of all cancer cases. This tumor, though, has sought out at least one famous victim. Charles Revson, the founder and controlling force of the Revlon cosmetics empire, died of pancreatic cancer in 1975.

The pancreas is a glandular structure, seven to ten inches long, that lies behind the stomach for most of its length. Digestive enzymes and the hormone insulin are made by the pancreas. The only major diseases to which the adult organ is susceptible are pancreatitis (an inflammation usually caused by too much drinking), diabetes mellitus, and cancer.

The cause of pancreatic cancer is unknown. There is no good evidence that pancreatitis, alcoholism, syphilis, or any other diseases, for that matter, predispose to tumor formation. But sex is important: men are affected three to four times as frequently as women, usually between the ages of thirty-five and seventy.

Charles Revson's case of pancreatic carcinoma is fairly typical. Revson's first characteristic symptom was jaundice, a yellowing of the skin caused by retention within the body of bile. After passing through the liver, bile normally is piped into the small bowel by the common bile duct. But Revson's pancreatic cancer grew large enough to obstruct the duct, thereby causing the bile to pass into the bloodstream and produce the disagreeable yellow skin hue. The diagnosis of pancreatic cancer was confirmed at surgery, but no biopsy of the tumor was taken for fear of creating an abnormal connection to other parts of the digestive tract. The blocked common bile duct was reconnected above the obstructed segment to correct the jaundice, and the patient was sent home.

Revson was aware that he was seriously ill, and he wanted to know just what his outlook was. The doctors, expecting his death within a short time, were quite candid. Knowing he must choose a successor to run his cosmetics empire, Revson tapped Michel Bergerac, the president of ITT Europe, whose French accent is said to be thicker than *creme fraiche.*

But Revson fooled the doctors. Six months after his first operation he was still alive, though complaining of severe abdominal pain, a common symptom in pancreatic cancer resulting from tumor growth into nearby nerves. A second operation was performed, and this time a small tumor specimen could be taken to confirm the diagnosis. In spite of the radiation therapy administered, the disease continued to progress, with death occurring on August 24, 1975.

Certain rare pancreatic tumors, islet cell tumors, cause symptoms much different from those Charles Revson had. A functioning islet cell tumor leads to an overproduction of the hormone insulin. Patients experience low blood sugar, fatigue, and weakness that can progress to staggering, lowered body temperature, and coma. These manifestations occur in intermittent attacks, most frequently in the morning before breakfast. The nonfunctioning tumors, also called Zollinger-Ellison tumors, elaborate a protein hormone, gastrin, that leads to overproduction of stomach acid and severe ulcer disease in some patients, an unmanageable watery diarrhea in others.

No specific test to positively identify pancreatic cancer exists, but its presence can be inferred in various ways. An upper GI series, the same X-ray examination used to diagnose stomach abnormalities, can sometimes show the presence of a mass in the region of the pancreas. A special flexible instrument, the fiberoptic duodenoscope, can be passed through the mouth and stomach into the small bowel to allow a tube to be inserted into the bile duct opening; a special iodine-containing liquid is then injected to allow the bile duct to be seen on an X-ray film. Long, thin tubes can be passed through an artery in the leg until they reach the blood vessels supplying the pancreas;

injection of another iodine-containing dye then allows these arteries to be seen on an X ray. The computerized axial tomographic (CAT) scanner, an exciting new instrument now revolutionizing medical diagnosis, actually allows X-ray pictures of the pancreas to be made and is said to be able to detect very small pancreatic tumors long before they first produce symptoms.

Surgery is the most widely employed curative procedure in pancreatic cancer, but the survival rate is dismal—less than 2 percent of patients alive after five years. Curative surgery can only be done on those pancreatic tumors that involve solely the head of the pancreas, that part of the organ closest to the midline of the body. The necessary treatment, the Whipple procedure, is one of the most extensive cancer operations ever devised, and a significant number of patients die from its aftereffects. Because of these poor results, better methods are being sought.

Radiotherapy seems to hold promise. In a recent study, Drs. John Haslam and Patrick Cavanaugh at Duke Medical School used high doses of external radiation to early pancreatic tumors. Instead of giving the treatments on consecutive days, as is usually done, the doctors broke the course of therapy into three two-week segments, each separated by two weeks. An amazing five-year survival rate of 20 percent was reported, and good symptomatic relief was achieved in many patients who could not be cured.

The treatment of islet cell tumors is exclusively surgical. The functioning tumors must be surgically excised. Zollinger-Ellison tumors require total removal of the stomach if ulcer disease is present. Some islet cell tumors turn out to be nonmalignant, and patients suffering them generally do well after surgery.

Liver Cancer

Cancer of the liver is relatively rare in the United States, making up roughly 2 percent of all cancer cases. This is not the situation among Orientals or the South African Bantu, where for reasons unknown the disease is much more common.

Men are affected six to ten times more frequently than women, and people usually contract the disease between the ages of sixty and seventy. While no specific causative agent has been implicated, four conditions are predisposing: liver cirrhosis, intestinal parasites, hemochromatosis, and industrial exposure to chemicals, most recently vinyl chloride.

Liver cirrhosis is a chronic disease in which the ordinarily smooth and well-formed liver is distorted by masses of fibrous tissue and nodules. Cirrhosis is known to most people because of its association with alcoholism or just plain too much drinking. Other less familiar causes are viral liver infections (hepatitis), malnutrition, heart failure, and syphilis. Cirrhosis is present in 70 percent of all patients with liver cancer; conversely, in one large study, about 5 percent of patients with cirrhosis had a coincidental liver cancer.

Intestinal parasites, especially those that spend most of their time in the liver, are closely related to the development of some liver cancers. *Clonorchis sinensis,* the Oriental liver fluke, has been observed in 15 percent of liver cancer cases occurring in Hong Kong. *Fasciola hepatica,* the sheep liver fluke, is seen associated with cases in sheep-raising countries.

Hemochromatosis is a rare disease in which abnormally large quantities of the iron-containing compounds ferritin and hemosiderin are deposited throughout the body. The usual patient, a man between the ages of thirty and fifty, has liver disease, diabetes, and brownish skin pigmentation. As these individuals age, liver cancer will develop in many of them.

Angiosarcoma of the liver is a very rare type of cancer, there being only twenty to twenty-five cases a year in the whole United States. The B. F. Goodrich Company was therefore alarmed to discover that, among workers in one of its factories where vinyl chloride was used, there had been one death from angiosarcoma of the liver in 1971 and two in 1973. These men had worked with vinyl chloride for fifteen to twenty-eight years. Two additional cases of this form of cancer have since been reported among vinyl chloride workers, one in the United States and one in Britain. Responsible firms are now warning their workers of the possible hazard and working to reduce atmospheric levels of gaseous vinyl chloride in the workplace.

The initial symptoms of liver cancer are rather nonspecific complaints: weakness, loss of appetite, abdominal fullness or bloating, and dull or aching upper abdominal pain. As the disease progresses, the liver enlarges, and a definite lump may be palpable in the abdomen. A great diagnostic aid at this point is the radioisotope liver scan.

To perform a liver scan, a compound containing the radioactive element technetium 99m is injected into a vein in the arm. The compound is taken up by cells within the liver almost immediately. By using an instrument called a rectilinear scanner, the radioactivity can be detected from outside the body and a good image of the liver can be produced on a piece of X-ray film. Tumors larger than an inch in size are readily detected by this method.

The final confirmation of the diagnosis of liver cancer is often made by biopsy, the removing of a small piece of tissue. This may be accomplished by means of a hollow needle inserted through the abdomen into the tumor. Ordinarily this procedure is accompanied by little pain and few complications. Biopsy is important because, if examination of the tumor shows it to have spread to the liver from elsewhere, rather than originating in the liver, curative treatment is usually not possible.

The definitive treatment for a liver cancer is surgical removal. And cure can only be effected if the tumor is solitary and localized with no evidence of distant spread. Radiation therapy is considered to be of little value here; the lesions are said not to be radiosensitive, and normal liver tissue tolerates radiation poorly. Some anticancer drugs are of help in relieving symptoms, notably the compounds methotrexate and 5-fluorouracil.

If the cancer is incurable, the course of the illness is generally rapid; most patients die within six months of diagnosis.

A few cases of long-term survival after surgery have been reported, but the overall five-year survival rate is less than 1 percent.

Cancer of the Gallbladder and Bile Ducts

The breakdown of red blood cells within the body produces the yellowish, oily liquid bile. Known to the ancients, so-called yellow bile and black bile were two of the four "humors" of medieval medicine and were felt to be responsible for a vile-tempered or bilious personality, as well as for certain diseases.

The body rids itself of bile by passing it through the liver. After a complex chemical alteration within the liver cells, the bile flows through an intricate network of bile ducts into the common bile duct and thence to the small bowel. On its way, much of the bile finds its way into a muscular, pouchlike storage reservoir, the gallbladder. Once merely an annoying waste product, the altered bile now aids in the digestion of fat; large quantities are liberated by the gallbladder after a fatty meal.

Cancer of the gallbladder is the sixth most common cancer of the digestive tract and accounts for 4 percent of all forms of cancer. Found three to four times more often in women, this cancer occurs most commonly around the age of seventy and is rare before age forty.

Gallbladder cancer has a very close relationship to other gallbladder disease. The increased incidence in women parallels the greater amount of gallbladder ailments in women. One per-cent of all patients operated on for acute inflammation of the gallbladder have cancer found at surgery. The incidence of gall-bladder cancer in patients with gallstones has been reported to be between 4 and 5 percent. And 98 percent of patients with cancer have associated gallstones. Even in guinea pigs, experi-mental gallbladder cancer has been produced by the insertion of sterile, hard stones.

Symptoms of gallbladder cancer may be confused with those of gallbladder inflammation, since the patient has often suffered numerous gallbladder attacks. Pain in the right upper part of the abdomen that becomes progressively more severe accompanies nausea and vomiting. Jaundice, a yellowing of the skin caused by bile retention, occurs in 60 percent of cases. In addition, loss of weight and appetite may have been noted. Presence of the disease is usually not confirmed until surgery, as there are no diagnostic tests that can reveal it.

The only hope for cure is complete surgical removal of the gallbladder. Because of early invasion of the liver, much of this organ must also often be removed. The tumor is said to be insensitive to radiation, and no drugs are known to be of value. The results of treatment are extremely poor, with less than 3 percent of patients surviving five years. Ninety percent of patients will die within the first year after the disease has been discovered.

Cancer of the bile ducts is rare, less than a third as common as gallbladder cancer. The disease is slightly more common in men than in women, and most patients are in their sixties or seventies. The principal symptoms are jaundice, pain, and weight loss. Some difficulty attends the diagnosis of this disease, which is usually only made at surgery. When the cancer occurs at the ampulla—the point where the common bile duct opens into the small bowel—surgery can produce a 33 percent five-year survival. But for other bile duct cancers, no cures can be obtained by any method.

6 Cancer of the Male Genital Tract and Urinary Tract

The Prostate and "Everyman's Cancer"

The prostate is a chestnut-shaped gland that lies at the base of the male bladder. Its function is the formation of semen within its recesses and expulsion by muscular contraction during ejaculation. But the prostate is also a great troublemaker. The enlargement of the gland that often occurs from middle age onward can reduce a once powerful stream of urine to a pathetic dribble. Urologists (surgeons who treat only urinary tract disorders) spend the bulk of their working days battling this pesky structure so that men of sixty can void like men of twenty.

Cancer of the prostate is the second most common malignancy in men over fifty, exceeded only by skin cancer. Doctors see thirty-eight thousand new cases each year and almost eighteen thousand deaths. The disease increases in incidence every year after age of sixty, and a much higher number of non-symptomatic cases are discovered only at autopsy. Because of its ubiquitous nature, Dr. Bernard Roswit, an eminent cancer specialist, has called this tumor "everyman's cancer." Sam Rayburn, one of the greatest Speakers of the House of Representatives, died of prostate cancer.

The cause of prostate cancer is unknown, and, unlike many other cancers, no predisposing factors have been discovered. Asian, African, and Latin American countries have far fewer cases than does the United States, which has the world's highest incidence. The low incidence rate in Japanese men contrasts with a much higher one for Japanese Americans. Prostatic enlargement, called hypertrophy, does not lead to greater susceptibility to prostate cancer.

Pioneering advances in prostate disease diagnosis and treatment were made early in this century by the urologist Dr. Hugh Hampton Young. So grateful was the legendary Diamond Jim Brady after being cured of a urinary obstruction by Dr. Young that the gambler built the Brady Urologic Institute at Johns Hopkins for him. Admirers and rivals both agreed that the organ that makes most men old made Hugh Young.

Dr. Young's classification of the initial symptoms of prostate cancer is still valid today. The urge to urinate frequently is most common; it is present in over two thirds of cases. Pain on urination is an early symptom in half the cases. Generalized pain, especially low back pain, occurs in a third of patients; this symptom was especially troubling to Sam Rayburn. Only rarely will inability to urinate (urinary retention) or blood in the urine be early symptoms.

Later in the disease, symptoms become more severe. Difficulty starting urination, unexplained bladder infections or urinary bleeding, inability to urinate, bone pain and anemia are commonly observed. But unlike other cancers that involve the skeleton, prostate cancer rarely causes bones to fracture.

Early diagnosis by a physician is made in two ways. One is rectal examination, which can reveal a small, hard nodule palpable within the prostate; one half of such nodules will be malignant.[1] Another is routine microscopic examination of tissue removed from an enlarged prostate to relieve urinary obstruction; such tissue often shows small areas of cancer. Most often this is adenocarcinoma (glandular cancer) and arises from prostatic glandular tissue: rarely the cancer is classified as a sarcoma because it has presumably developed from connective tissue.

Once prostate cancer is detected or suspected, a whole battery of tests is used to verify the presence and extent of the disease.

---

1. Rectal self-examination, a new method, is described earlier.

If the first sign is a nodule palpated on rectal exam, a piece of suspect tissue may be removed by means of a needle biopsy taken through the rectum. Acid and alkaline phosphatase, two enzymes found in the blood, will be present in abnormally high concentration in two-thirds of patients. Metastatic deposits of cancer in the skeleton can be seen on X-ray examination. But an even more sensitive method of detecting such deposits is a bone scan.

During a bone scan, a radioactive compound, technetium polyphosphate or technetium diphosphonate, is injected into a vein. For reasons unknown, these particular chemicals are taken up by the bones. The radioactivity may be detected with an instrument called a whole body scanner, and a photographic film image made of the entire skeleton. Regions involved by tumor will show up as dark spots.

Since the days of Dr. Hugh Hampton Young, radical prostatectomy—a complete removal of the prostate and part of the bladder—has been the only way to cure prostate cancer. When this operation is performed on a healthy male of less than seventy years of age without evidence of cancer spread, the patient has a 50 percent chance of surviving five years. Such patients comprise about 10 percent of all prostate cancer cases.

But radical prostatectomy has unpleasant characteristic complications besides those associated with surgery in general. Impotence always occurs because of surgical destruction of the erection-stimulating nerve network around the prostate. From 5 to 15 percent of patients will become completely incontinent (unable to hold urine) due to surgical disturbance of muscular sphincters that normally act as valves. The only recourse is a lifetime of wearing a tube around the penis with a bag strapped to one leg to catch the urine.

The use of radiation therapy instead of surgery has proved to be a good method of circumventing unpleasant surgical complications. Dr. Malcolm Bagshaw at Stanford has treated a large series of localized prostate cancer cases exclusively with radiation therapy. Sixty percent of the patients survived five years.

No instances of incontinence after therapy were reported. An additional bonus was that potency was maintained in 75 percent of the cases. Even though some men brag and others lie, this figure is still quite impressive.

Once prostate cancer has spread to the bones or other parts of the body, cure is no longer possible. In these advanced cases, radiation therapy and hormonal therapy can provide great relief from pain.

Radiation therapy may be administered in two ways. The rays produced by cobalt sixty, a linear accelerator, or some other external X-ray source may be beamed to single tender areas. Or if many painful points are present, radioactive phosphorus-32 is injected into the body through a vein, often reducing discomfort considerably as the compound is taken up by the individual lesions.

Hormonal therapy of prostate carcinoma represents one of the great advances in modern medicine. Dr. Charles Huggins was awarded the Nobel Prize for discovery of this valuable technique. Dramatic results can be obtained in patients who have widespread disease and bone pain. Evidence of bone lesions may disappear, and within four to six weeks the prostate frequently shrinks to its normal size. Unfortunately, some men refuse hormonal therapy because of the procedures involved.

The first step is castration to prevent production of the tumor-stimulating male hormone testosterone. After the good effects of this procedure wear off, estrogen, the female hormone, must be administered. But along with pain relief, estrogen stimulates breast development and causes considerable breast tenderness. Small doses of radiation to both breasts prior to treatment can avert this complication. Unfortunately, estrogen also causes death from heart disease. This regrettable combination—the relief of pain but the shortening of life—now seems avoidable by giving reduced doses of estrogen.

Urinary Bladder Cancer

At the bottom of the pelvic cavity sits the urinary bladder, a muscular, membranous sac. A young man is conscious of his bladder only because it puts a constraint on the amount of time he may remain seated in a movie or make uninterrupted love. Young women are somewhat more aware of their bladders when a "honeymoon" infection occurs after intercourse. But the aging bladder may fall prey to a much more serious condition—cancer.

Bladder cancer is the most frequent malignant tumor of the entire urinary tract, doubtless due to a host of environmental factors. As early as 1906, workers in the aniline dye factories of the German Empire were observed to contract bladder cancer with alarming frequency. Studies of these cases, performed with customary Teutonic thoroughness, revealed that the length of dye exposure varied considerably, sometimes being as long as forty years. The chemical agents beta napthylamine and 4-amino diphenyl were found to be the culprits.

Cigarette smoking is another factor that plays a role in bladder cancer because of the tar contained in the smoke. Chronic infections, bladder stones, and the parasite *schistosoma hematobium* are often involved in a special type of bladder malignancy, the squamous cell tumor.

Most commonly, cancer of the bladder's first symptom is blood in the urine, found in 75 percent of all early cases. The bleeding characteristically occurs at intervals and this can delay diagnosis since the patient may pass off the abnormality as trivial and not bother to consult his physician. But blood in the urine is always a serious sign, one never to be disregarded.

Bladder irritability producing the urge to urinate, and pain on urination are present in about a third of the cases. As the disease progresses, these symptoms tend to increase in severity. Dr. Hugh Jewett, an eminent Johns Hopkins urologist, tells of one old gentleman who loved to golf but was annoyed by his increasingly frequent and urgent desire to urinate while on the links. After his golfing partners began to chuckle at his repeated need to relieve himself behind trees and bushes, the man finally went to his physician and then to Dr. Jewett, who confirmed the diagnosis of bladder tumor.

This diagnosis is usually not difficult to make. Examination of the urine under a microscope will show the presence of small numbers of red blood cells invisible to the unaided eye. A special X-ray examination, the intravenous pyelogram (IVP), allows the whole urinary tract, including the bladder, to be seen; although ordinarily invisible on X-ray film, this structure can be visualized after injecting into an arm vein an iodine-containing liquid that is excreted by the kidneys. A tubular optical device, the cystoscope, can be inserted through the penile or vulvar opening into the bladder to observe abnormalities directly. Pieces of tumor can be removed through this instrument for microscopic analysis.

When the tumor is superficial (a papilloma), a burning wire can be inserted through a cystoscope to remove it. The hot wire is used both to cut and to control bleeding from the cut surface. Of course, the advantage here is that major surgery is avoided. A complete cure of slowly growing papillomas can often be achieved in this way, and even if there should be regrowth later, the same technique can be used again.

But fast-growing, more highly malignant tumors present a bigger problem. The enlarging cancer permeates deeply into the muscle of the bladder, making complete removal with the hot wire all but impossible. Here there is some controversy as to what form of treatment is best.

Sometimes just the tumor and an adequate margin of bladder wall can be cut out, a procedure called segmental resection. If a cure can be achieved, the patient will be left with a diminished bladder capacity but at least still alive and otherwise reasonably well. Unfortunately, though, some segmental resections fail, and other tumors are just too large for this treatment. What then?

Two alternatives are left: total removal of the bladder (total cystectomy) or high-dose radiation therapy. Total cystectomy is a difficult procedure at best. Closure of the wound itself is not easy, and urine must be diverted through a loop of disconnected small bowel into a plastic bag worn on the abdomen for the remainder of the patient's life. High-dose radiation therapy is easier to tolerate, since if the patient survives he will at least be able to urinate normally, although he may continue to be troubled by some bladder inflammation and diminished capacity. The low five-year survival rate from both surgery and radiotherapy, running in the 25 percent range, has led urologists such as Dr. George Prout of the Massachusetts General Hospital to opt for radiation in most cases. According to Dr. Prout, both techniques are equally bad, but at least radiotherapy may often be less disabling in the long run.

Testicular Cancer

Cancer of the testicle is one of the rarer malignancies in men, representing 1 percent of all cancer cases. The disease is primarily one of young men, with the greatest number of cases found between the ages of thirty and thirty-four. For reasons that are unclear, Negroes—especially the Bantu and the Cape Colored in South Africa—are rarely affected.

Testicular cancer is especially common in the condition called cryptochidism. Ordinarily the testes develop within the abdominal cavity during intrauterine life but descend into the scrotum as the infant matures. Some men's testicles never make the whole trip, however, and remain suspended along the normal route. Between 5 and 20 percent of these cases may develop a cancer.

A blow to the testicle is reported by as many as 10 percent of testicular cancer patients. In one case, a man told of having his testicle stomped on by his young son three months before a cancer had been discovered. Most urologists feel, though, that trauma is not a causal factor; instead, it merely serves to call attention to the presence of a tumor.

Few symptoms attend the early development of testicular cancer. Sometimes there may be simply a sensation of discomfort due to the weight of the tumor. Testicular sensitivity may also decrease. A young man may first go to his doctor after discovering a testicular lump while examining himself in the shower. But a urologist's letter to the *Journal of the American Medical Association* a few years ago complained that too few men examine themselves; testicular lumps are more often first palpated by a lover.

Once a lesion has been identified, an X-ray examination of the urinary tract (intravenous pyelogram) will be done to determine whether tumor has spread to the abdomen. A chest film quickly reveals any cancer within the lungs. The patient's chance to survive after adequate surgery can be estimated by evidence of tumor spread and also by the type of cell comprising the lesion.

The most favorable tumor type, occurring in 40 percent of cases, is the seminoma; 98 percent of men with early lesions can be expected to survive five years. Democratic Senator Frank Church of Idaho is one such survivor. Seminomas that have spread to the lymph nodes of the abdomen or even to the lungs are exquisitely sensitive to radiation and can be cured in many cases. Less curable are the embryonal carcinoma and teratoma, and worst of all is the choriocarcinoma. Unlike choriocarcinoma of the uterus, testicular choriocarcinoma cannot be cured with the drug methotrexate.

A very rare testicular growth is the interstitial cell tumor. The interstitial cells (also called leydig cells) manufacture the male hormone testosterone. Commonly occurring in boys between ages five and ten, interstitial cell tumors cause prococious sexual and body development, turning a second grader into a so-called infant Hercules, who is often first brought to the doctor after he has been exhibiting sexually precocious behavior. Fortunately, few interstitial cell tumors are malignant, and cure can be effected merely by removing the involved testicle.

Cancer of the Kidney

Of all human cancers, 1 to 2 percent occur in the kidney. This year 6,800 adults will die of kidney cancer, while another 11,400 new cases will be discovered. The average age at the time of diagnosis is between forty-five and sixty. Eighty percent of the tumors will be adenocarcinoma (derived from glandular tissue and also called hypernephroma), which afflict men twice as often as women. Another 15 percent of tumors grow from the renal pelvis—that part of the kidney that serves as a collecting cistern for urine—and here men and women are equally susceptible. No causative factors for kidney cancer are known.

The most common sign of kidney cancer is the appearance of blood in the urine (hematuria), an early warning in 70 percent of cases. Despite the dramatic nature of urinary blood, patients delay on the average twenty-three months before consulting a physician. Even when pain is present, fourteen months usually elapse before the doctor is visited. By then the cancer will have spread to other parts of the body in 37 percent of cases. The moral to this sad tale: blood in the urine is a serious indicator of disease and should never be ignored.

A few diagnostic procedures can be used to document the presence of a kidney cancer, though unfortunately none is practical as an early screening method. Microscopic examination of the urine occasionally reveals red blood cells. Intravenous pyelography (IVP), the X-ray test used to visualize the urinary tract, can show the presence of a mass distorting the normal kidney shape. Ultrasound devices, which use high-frequency sound waves, are capable of forming an image of the kidney lesion to disclose whether a benign, fluid-filled cyst or a cancer has caused the patient's problem; the new technique, computerized axial tomographic (CAT) scanning, accomplishes this imaging even better. The most definitive diagnostic method to date is the selective renal arteriogram, requiring the passing of a long thin tube through a leg artery into the kidney. A special liquid is then instilled through the tube, allowing the whole kidney to be clearly seen on X ray.

Surgery offers the only hope for cure of kidney cancer. The entire kidney must be removed if hypernephroma is present. If the tumor has grown from the renal pelvis, the ureter (the muscular tube that conducts urine from the kidney to the bladder) must also be cut out. If the surgeon thinks that some tumor has been left behind after operation, radiation therapy may be employed.

Long-term survival rates after kidney cancer are abysmally low. If the tumors are detected early, ten-year survival runs between 15 and 30 percent. But in more advanced cases, ten-year survival can be as low as 5 percent. Cancer rarely occurs within the ureter itself. But when it does, men are affected twice as often as women, and the most common sign, again, is blood in the urine. Sometimes surgery can be used for cure, and radiation therapy is administered to advanced cases. But survival here is worse than for kidney tumors: less than 10 percent of all treated patients live five years.

Cancer of the Penis

In the continental United States, penile cancer is one of the more uncommon forms of malignancy. Circumcision appears to prevent this tumor if performed in infancy and for this reason, Jews are practically never afflicted. Moslems, who are ritually circumcised between the ages of three and fourteen, have a higher incidence. Puerto Ricans and blacks have the largest number of cases.

The cancer may appear as an ulcer or sore on the penis, or as an enlarging, solid, cauliflowerlike mass. As the condition progresses, spontaneous bleeding and malodorous infection are often noted. Lumps in the groin develop, the result of tumor spread to the lymph nodes in this region.

When an early, small lesion is present, the involved portion of the penis may be amputated for cure. Quite understandably, this form of treatment is shunned by younger patients. For these individuals, radiation therapy with cobalt sixty offers an acceptable alternative; 90 percent should survive five years. When lymph nodes are involved the survival rate drops, but the condition is still far from hopeless. Drs. A. Taihefer and J. Courtial at the Fondation Curie in France report a 23 percent five-year survival in such cases.

7 Skin Cancer

Cancer of the skin is one of the most frequent forms of cancer—19 percent of all cancer in men, 11 percent of all cancer in women. Doctors estimate that 40 to 50 percent of people who live to be sixty-five will have at least one skin cancer. Skin cancer is also the most common second cancer; a person who has had one type of malignancy has a 50 to 60 percent chance of developing a subsequent tumor, usually a skin cancer.

Fortunately, skin cancer is very curable. Because the skin is so completely exposed to view, small lesions are usually detected earlier than in the colon, for example. Small lesions also lend themselves to good cosmetic results after treatment. Better than 90 percent of all skin cancer cases should survive five years after therapy, the only exception being malignant melanoma, a tumor that develops from a pigmented mole. An even higher percentage of cases could be prevented, however, if one harmful practice were stopped: sun bathing.

Many people believe that lying in the sun is healthy. After all, what looks better than a good suntan? But tans have not always been in fashion. In *Gone with the Wind,* Scarlett O'Hara's young lady friends protected their milk white complexions with large bonnets and parasols. When Scarlett announced she would attend a garden party in a brief dress, Mammy reacted swiftly: "No, you ain'. It ain' fittin fer mawnin'. You kain show yo' buzzum befo' three o'clock an' dat dress ain' got no neck an'

no sleeves. An' you'll git freckled sho as you born, an' Ah ain'
figgerin' on you gittin' freckled affer all de buttermilk Ah been
puttin' on you all dis winter, bleachin' dem freckles you got at
Savannah settin' on de beach. Ah sho gwine speak ter yo' Ma
'bout you."

The suntan craze came in during the 1920s with the enormous
popularity of Douglas Fairbanks, and it has remained the most
enduring legacy of the Jazz Age. Ironically, Fairbanks came by
the look accidentally, as he later related:

"I was so dark . . . my mother was ashamed of me. When all
the neighbors came around to look at the new baby, Mother
would say, 'Oh, I don't want to disturb him now—he's asleep
and I'd rather not.' "

But during the highly successful runs of *The Mark of Zoro,
Robin Hood,* and *The Black Pirate,* his dark skin became one
of the actor's trademarks, and Fairbanks fans flocked into the
sun in droves to attain the same swarthy appearance. These and
other victims of overexposure to sunlight continue to contract
skin cancers at a frightening rate.

The amount of sun exposure is directly related to the frequency with which cancer develops. Individuals occupied in out-
door work, such as farmers and sailors, tend to get lesions on
uncovered areas. The greater amount of sunshine in the tropics
may be responsible for high skin cancer rates of inhabitants.
But in addition to sun, there are other causative elements.

Sexual and racial factors play a large role in determining
susceptibility to skin cancer. Men are afflicted more often than
women. Those with a ruddy complexion—Scandinavians and
north Germans, for example—seem to develop more skin cancers after chronic sun exposure than do individuals with coarser,
darker skin. Arabs, South American Indians, and blacks are
only slightly vulnerable to skin cancers. Scientists once believed
that dark skin conferred an evolutionary advantage by permit-
ting survival in sunny climates. But recently, nutritionists have
theorized that light skin has its own advantages, allowing vitamin D synthesis in the skin in parts of the world where sunlight
is more sparse.

A rare oversensitivity to the sun's rays leads to a condition known as xeroderma pigmentosum and to the development of multiple cancers of the skin in children. Sufferers from this hereditary disorder must protect themselves from all sunlight with the greatest care. And families of these patients should be thoroughly investigated to discover additional cases so that measures can be instituted to prevent cancers from forming.

Contact with or ingestion of certain chemical agents can lead to skin cancer. Arsenic is most frequently implicated, especially in factory workers and in syphilis patients treated with arsenical compounds before the advent of penicillin. Tar and pitch are also causative agents; in fact, the first carcinogenic material ever identified, soot, was described in the eighteenth century by an English physician, Dr. Percival Pott, who recognized it as the cause of cancer of the scrotum in chimney sweeps.

Burn scars and sinus tracts are susceptible to cancer of the skin. In burns, cancers may arise twenty to forty years after the injury, usually from chronically ulcerated tissue within the scar. Chronic bone infection (osteomyelitis) leads to openings (sinus tracts) forming between the bone and the skin surface, from which pus continually drains. As in burn scars, cancer tends to occur in sinus tracts many years after the tracts originally appear. Today, fortunately, antibiotics have made chronic osteomyelitis a condition doctors seldom see.

Most skin cancers are one of two types: squamous cell carcinomas or basal cell carcinomas. The squamous cell lesion is scaly and elevated, with an irregular border and a shallow, non-healing central ulcer. The basal cell lesion is similar but tends to burrow more deeply into the skin, thus attaining the nickname of "rodent ulcer." Squamous cell cancers can metastasize and begin to grow in other parts of the body; basal cell cancers cannot.

Definitive diagnosis of skin cancer is made by biopsy—removal of the lesion and microscopic examination. If small, the tumor can be totally excised for study; larger tumors may have a portion removed. No other diagnostic maneuvers are usually required.

The two standard methods for curing skin cancers are surgery and radiation therapy. Surgery is ordinarily required for any tumors that invade bone or cartilage. These are difficult to cure with radiation, and the cartilage is sometimes left permanently damaged by the X rays. Small tumors can be easily treated surgically. But what if the tumor arises from a cosmetically important region, such as the lip? Of course, the surgeon can still excise the tumor, but that lip will never look the same again. Radiation therapy, on the other hand, can produce an equally effective cure while preserving perfectly the cosmetic appearance. The same can be said for tumors of any part of the face where a surgical scar would be highly unsightly.

In the past few years, certain drugs and chemical agents have been found effective against skin cancer. Drug therapy is indicated when there is not one tumor but many. The compound nitrogen mustard can be applied as a cream to kill tumor cells directly. A more elegant method involves the application of dinitrochlorobenzene (DNCB) cream, which excites an immune reaction and causes the patient's body to destroy the cancer cells as though they were foreign invaders.

Special Forms of Skin Cancer

Unlike squamous and basal cell carcinomas, the ordinary forms of skin cancer, three special forms—mycosis fungoides, Kaposi's sarcoma, and malignant melanoma—are more difficult to deal with. None of these is derived from the regular epithelial cells that make up the skin, and all are relatively rare.

Mycosis fungoides is a malignant skin condition with cells that look very similar to those found in leukemia. Raised skin plaques, frequently itchy, continue to form over many years; these are very sensitive to X rays and can be helped greatly with radiation therapy. Death comes in some cases when the disease spreads to involve other organs.

Kaposi's sarcoma is another very slowly growing form of cancer arising from blood vessels. For reasons unknown, Italian and Jewish men are most commonly affected. Purplish or reddish nodules that tend to increase in size are first noted on the lower legs and feet but eventually spread to other parts of the skin. Like mycosis fungoides, the lesions of Kaposi's sarcoma are very sensitive to radiation, but they may eventually cause death by extending into other organs.

Malignant melanoma is a unique and important form of skin cancer, quite different from the others just discussed. It arises from the cells within a mole or nevus, a brown-pigmented lesion found in the skin of almost everyone. Despite its universality, the nevus cell is something of a mystery. What is its function? Where does it come from? Some researchers have suggested that a form of nerve cell may be related to the nevus cell, but no one is certain.

The average Caucasian has fifteen pigmented skin moles, the average Negro, two. The chance of a mole's becoming cancerous is one in a million, which accounts for malignant melanoma's relative rarity—1.2 percent of all forms of cancer. American Negroes seem to be affected more commonly than African Negroes, probably because of their white racial heritage. The peak incidence occurs between the ages of fifty and sixty, especially in light-complected individuals. The head and neck are most frequently involved, followed by the legs. Exposure to sunlight appears to play a causative role, as does chronic irritation, for example by a belt or brassiere strap.

A melanoma appears as a brown or black spot that usually has grown from a preexisting mole. As the lesion enlarges, it often shows the following changes: irregular intensity of color, focal loss of color, expansive growth, ulceration, blistering, redness, or soreness. A rare form of melanoma, amelanotic melanoma, contains no brown pigment at all.

The treatment is surgical excision, if the lesion is small enough, and the removal of any lymph nodes that may be close by. Radiation therapy is usually of no value. Recently, promising results have been obtained with BCG, a bacterial vaccine used for many years to immunize against tuberculosis. When injected into the skin lesions, the BCG provokes a powerful immune response, causing even distant tumor to regress or disappear. Five-year survival has been enhanced by this technique. Survival results for malignant melanoma are considerably worse than for ordinary skin cancer. Seventy percent of patients with superficial lesions less than an inch in diameter survive five years. People with larger tumors that have not spread to other sites have a 45 percent five-year survival rate. But if lymph nodes are involved, the figure drops to 16.2 percent, and no patient with distant lesions, in the liver or brain for example, can be expected to recover. One such unfortunate victim may well have been the thirty-second president of the United States, Franklin D. Roosevelt.

Great men should have an autopsy, and the findings should be made public, so that natural curiosity or unwarranted speculation may be dispelled. In the absence of authoritative information, private inquiries inevitably disclose facts that were previously unknown and that become the basis of mystery and legend. Inquiries of this nature, lacking information from the Roosevelt family, certainly implicate melanoma as a cause of FDR's death, as Dr. Hugh L'Etang has pointed out in his book, *The Pathology of Leadership.*

An American physician, Dr. F. M. Massie, noticed a pigmented mole above Roosevelt's left eyebrow that did not appear in photographs after 1943. At a medical meeting in Saint Louis, Missouri, in 1949, surgeons from the Walter Reed Army Hospital, Washington, D.C., presented a paper on the treatment of malignant melanoma. All the slides and specimens shown had a serial number, with one exception. This was a section of brain with a large metastatic deposit of melanoma in the right hemisphere. It merely bore a date: 14 April 1945. The fact that this was the day on which Roosevelt's body arrived in Washington from Warm Springs, Georgia, makes this observation rather more than a mere coincidence.

8 Leukemias and Lymphomas

Leukemias

In 1845 Rudolf Virchow, the great German pathologist, performed an autopsy on a fifty-year-old female cook and found a condition he labelled "white blood" because of the great predominance of "colorless" cells. He called the affliction leukemia and was later able to recognize two distinct forms. Previously, leukemia had been misdiagnosed as anemia, and patients were treated by having them drink blood. Another physician, John Hughes Bennett, independently discovered leukemia at about the same time, but Virchow published the first detailed description in his now-classic textbook, *Cellular Pathology*. His hypothesis—now known to be correct—was that all cells, including leukemia cells, were formed by division from other cells, *omnis cellula a cellula,* a radical departure from the then-accepted theory of free formation of cells from "cytoblastema." By the time of Virchow's death after a fall from a Berlin streetcar in 1902, his ideas were recognized as "a flight out of Egypt" for medical theory.

As Virchow realized, the leukemias are a group of diseases primarily involving two types of tissue, lymphatic and myelogenous. Lymphatic tissue, found in small, round clusters called lymph nodes, is spread through the body in structures resembling chains. It provides a form of immunity called humoral immunity, by making antibodies that damage invading organisms. Lymphatic tissue also produces blood cells called lymphocytes. Myelogenous tissue is present in the bone marrow and produces most of the cells found in the blood. Occasionally a few immature cells in either lymphatic or myelogenous tissue lose the ability to respond to forces normally regulating their maturation and proliferation. If the cells are lymphocytes, a lymphocytic leukemia is the result. If cells of the myelogenous tissue go sour, a variety of different leukemias can develop: stem cell leukemia, monocytic leukemia, myelogenous leukemia, erythroleukemia, plasmacytic leukemia, or the rarest of all, mast cell leukemia.

Although leukemia has been an uncommon disease in the past, its incidence is now increasing, especially among older individuals. William Wellman, the tough, carousing Hollywood director-writer, whose films *Wings, The Public Enemy,* and *The Ox Bow Incident* brought him world acclaim, was a recent victim at age seventy-nine. For reasons that are unclear, the disorder is two and a half times more common in blacks than in whites. Exposure to radiation definitely is predisposing, as evidenced by increased incidence in the survivors of Hiroshima and Nagasaki and in radiologists and other persons occupationally exposed to X rays.

Contact with certain chemicals and drugs can produce leukemia in animals and probably affects humans similarly. A study of the deaths of members of the American Chemical Society revealed an abnormally large number of leukemias, presumably because of chemists' frequent inhalation of volatile organic solvents such as benzene. The use of certain drugs—phenylbutazone for the treatment of gout, arsenical compounds for syphilis therapy, and the antibiotic chloramphenicol—has been observed to be related to the subsequent development of leukemia.

Heredity plays an important role in leukemia. The disease is especially common in a number of genetic disorders:

Mongolism (Down's syndrome) is caused by an extra chromosome; most such children are born to older mothers. Such a child is severely mentally retarded and has the slanted "Oriental" eyes for which the condition is named. Besides increased incidence of leukemia, congenital deformities of the heart and digestive tract are also common.

Franconi's anemia is a rare disorder in which there is too little blood-producing bone marrow. Accompanying this primary abnormality are multiple defects within the skeleton and urinary tract. Although it is usually fatal in childhood, survivors tend to die of hemorrhage, infection, or leukemia.

Klinefelter's syndrome, a relatively common genetic abnormality, occurs once in every four hundred live male births. As in mongolism, an extra chromosome is at fault, in this case an extra sex chromosome, the X chromosome. Affected men are tall, have very small testes, and usually are mentally retarded.

Additionally, there is a marked increase in frequency of leukemia in the identical twin of a leukemia patient. No such increase has ever been found in spouses of leukemia patients.

Myelogenous Leukemia

Acute myelogenous leukemia (AML) occurs with nearly equal frequency throughout life, but a bit more often after the age of forty. Men are afflicted slightly more often than women.

The major manifestations of AML are the result of the absence of normal blood cells. The normal blood-producing cells of the marrow are forced out and replaced by leukemic cells. Patients complain of pallor, fatigue, shortness of breath and increased thumping of the heart.

Other manifestations a physician can find are anemia and infections, such as skin abscesses, laryngitis, or pneumonia. The reduction in blood platelets—special cells needed for clotting—leads to abnormal bleeding from the gums, stomach, and urinary tract. Red spots on the skin that do not blanch on pressure, called petechiae or purpura, result from the same bleeding tendency. The spleen often enlarges to such a degree that awareness of an abdominal mass first brings the patient to a physician.

Making a laboratory diagnosis of leukemia is usually not difficult. An ordinary complete blood count performed on a blood sample from an arm vein can be sufficient. In addition, a piece of bone marrow can easily be sucked out by inserting a needle through the base of the spine into the sacrum. Microscopic examination will reveal the degree of marrow replacement by leukemic cells.

The treatment of acute myelogenous leukemia, as well as other forms, rests on two important premises: (1) that there are two competing cell lines present in the bone marrow—a leukemic cell line and a normal or nearly normal one, and (2) that a profound suppression of the leukemic marrow is required to allow the opportunity for a return of normal blood cell formation.

Several types of drugs have proved useful in reducing the number of leukemic marrow cells: cytosine arabinoside, mercaptopurine, thioguanine, and others. But because the level of normal blood cells is also reduced, transfusions of blood are inevitably required during therapy. The average survival of untreated patients is only two months, but intensive therapy has increased this to thirteen months by inducing remissions in the disease; during these periods, the patient appears and feels normal. Some remissions have even lasted so long as to be classified as cures.

Chronic myelogenous leukemia has a slower and more insidious onset than does AML, and some patients without symptoms are discovered during a routine medical examination. An abnormal chromosome, the Philadelphia chromosome, is present in the disordered white blood cells, the only specific and consistent genetic abnormality ever identified in leukemia. The antileukemic agent Busulfan is particularly effective in ameliorating the symptoms of the disease, though the mean survival time of three and a half years remains unaltered.

Acute Lymphocytic Leukemia

Cancers are the second most frequent cause of death in children, and acute lymphocytic leukemia is the most common of these cancers. Every year six individuals are affected per hundred thousand, with the highest incidence between the ages of three and four years. In some cases the leukemia is present at birth. It is rarely seen after age fifteen, and affects boys slightly more often than girls.

Before the late 1940s, acute leukemia in children was an incurable and rapidly fatal disease. Young patients were treated with blood transfusions and then sent home to await death in a few months from massive hemorrhage or overwhelming infection. Determined to find a better treatment, Dr. Sidney Farber, a professor of pathology at Harvard, embarked on his now historic search for an effective antileukemic drug.

In 1944, one researcher had reported success administering the concentrated vitamin folic acid to inhibit the growth of certain tumors in mice. This work suggested to Farber that chemical derivatives of folic acid might be effective in the treatment of human cancer. But to his surprise, he found that the leukemic process was actually accelerated by these compounds. These data suggested that growth of leukemic cells might be arrested if they were deprived of folic acid. At Farber's request, a series of drugs that blocked the action of folic acid were synthesized, and these were subsequently found capable of altering and disrupting the metabolism of leukemic cells.

In the winter of 1947, Farber administered aminopterin, one of the antifolates, to a critically ill child with acute leukemia. The disease dramatically regressed. Although the patient died soon afterwards, Farber had proved that a drug could induce a complete but temporary remission in a child with acute leukemia. And though temporary remission was not cure, it was now possible, as Farber said, "to prolong life, and this can be a good life." Farber's historic discovery of aminopterin not only lengthened the lives of many children with acute leukemia, but also brought about a new form of cancer management—chemotherapy, the treatment of cancer with drugs.

Shortly after Farber's achievement, other anticancer medications began to appear, such as methotrexate, first used in the treatment of childhood and acute leukemias and later for choriocarcinoma, a uterine tumor. Farber himself contributed yet another agent against childhood cancer when his experiments with highly toxic antibiotics revealed that actinomycin D was of value in the therapy of a kidney cancer of children called a Wilms' tumor.

One anticancer agent, nitrogen mustard, was found in a curious way. During the First World War, mustard gas was a fearsome new weapon. Soldiers in the trenches tried to detect its approach by keeping canaries nearby. So sensitive were these little birds that they dropped dead with the first whiff, warning the men to put on their gas masks. Unfortunately, in spite of this unusual biologic early warning system, many soldiers perished. Autopsy examinations revealed that, besides the severe lung damage, there was tremendous shrinkage of lymph nodes and lymphatic tissue. Years later, researchers looking for new anticancer drugs came across these old results and realized that, if injected into a vein, the mustard might be effective against lymphatic cancers. Nitrogen mustard, as we now know the compound, is today a widely used cancer-fighting drug.

The most frequent manifestations of acute lymphocytic leukemia result from the reduction of normal blood cells and the tissue accumulation of leukemic cells. Normally active children first begin to fatigue easily and feel unwell, then suffer fever and nasal, gum, or skin bleeding. Enlarged lymph nodes can be palpated as hard, rounded lumps under the skin. Arthritislike joint pains and bone pains are very often noticed. As the name of the disease implies, the onset is very rapid, much like a cold; most patients have symptoms less than six weeks before a physician is consulted.

As in other forms of leukemia, the diagnosis is not difficult to confirm. A blood count performed on a blood sample removed from a vein is frequently sufficient. During treatment, small samples of bone marrow are examined periodically to judge response to therapy.

Treatment of acute lymphocytic leukemia, like treatment of all leukemias, is based on the premise that reducing the number of leukemic cells will allow regrowth of the normal blood cells. This can be accomplished without producing the bone marrow suppression so common in other forms of leukemia therapy, since acute lymphocytic leukemia calls are so drug-sensitive. Three phases of treatment are generally recognized: the induction phase, the maintenance phase, and the intensification phase. During the induction or initial phase, two agents are used: the drug vincristine and the antiinflammatory steroid drug prednisone. These two compounds have very little effect on the normal blood-forming cells; as a result, rapid return to normal blood production is usually seen during the early treatment period, and so this period is less hazardous than in acute myelogenous leukemia. During the maintenance phase, continued drug therapy with such agents as methotrexate and 6-mercaptopurine tends to prolong the disease remissions. When a remission has been induced but is not complete, an intensification phase, in which greater amounts of medications are administered, can often bring on a fuller remission. But treatment with drugs by mouth is not adequate to destroy leukemic cells in some parts of the body, especially in the nervous system.

Nature has cleverly contrived, after eons of evolution, to protect the central nervous system at all cost. Among a whole bushel of ingenious protective devices is the blood-brain barrier, which allows no chemicals to enter the brain or spinal cord save a few simple and essential molecules such as oxygen, and glucose. As churches acted as sanctuaries during the Middle Ages for those pursued by the law, so the nervous system serves to shield some leukemic cells from pursuit by potent drugs in the blood. Fortunately, ever resourceful physicians have managed to circumvent this difficulty in two ways. High-energy external radiation, as with cobalt sixty, can be given to the whole brain and spinal cord to kill the malignant cells. Or after a spinal tap performed with a special long needle, methotrexate can be introduced directly into the spinal fluid; doctors call this intrathecal methotrexate.

In addition to drug therapy and radiation therapy, other adjuncts are being tried. Bone marrow transplants to replenish blood cells have been effective in some cases, but the same problems that plague the more dramatic heart and kidney transplants—rejection and infection—are also in evidence here. Efforts are now being made to stimulate the patient's own immune system to attack the leukemic cells by administering BCG antituberculosis vaccine or irradicated leukemic cells. Transfusions of blood cells during this period can strengthen the patient and confer some increased protection against infection.

Treatment of acute lymphocytic leukemia in children has proved to be one of the great triumphs of modern cancer therapy. Once this disease meant death within a few months. Now half of all patients are living five years. Longer and longer survivals have been reported with increasing frequency, and a small proportion of children remain disease-free indefinitely, even after cessation of drug therapy; however, infection during remission remains a serious problem and causes about 15 percent of deaths. Doctors worry that long-term drug therapy may have its own hazards, possibly inducing other tumors later in life, but thus far no such complications have been observed.

Preleukemia

Several nonmalignant blood disorders can terminate in leukemia. These are referred to by various terms: preleukemia, herald state of leukemia, or refractory anemia. Most commonly, patients have a severe anemia that won't respond to any form of treatment. Recent studies of the blood cells of such individuals reported by Dr. D. W. Golde in the *New England Journal of Medicine* have revealed definite differences between these cells and normal cells. But usually preleukemia is a diagnosis made in hindsight.

Chronic Lymphocytic Leukemia

Unlike acute lymphocytic leukemia, chronic lymphocytic leukemia is a disease of older people, usually between the ages of fifty and seventy. Men are affected three times as often as women. The onset is gradual and insidious, with increasing weakness, fatigue, and loss of appetite. Enlarged lymph nodes can be palpated as hard, rounded lumps under the skin. In a quarter of patients the disorder is first detected on a routine blood examination. Chronic lymphocytic leukemia is often a relatively benign condition. Although it is progressive, patients may be afflicted for many years without symptoms. And treatment with drugs and radiation can cause all evidence of the disease to disappear. Although the average survival time after symptoms appear is three to four years, many individuals live much longer, often to die of another, totally unrelated condition.

Lymphomas

Hodgkin's Disease

Enlargement of the spleen and lymph nodes as part of a chronic and eventually fatal disease was identified by the great English physician of London's Guy's Hospital, Thomas Hodgkin. Although Hodgkin himself believed that many other "morbid anatomists" of the day had actually observed the physical changes he described in the course of performing autopsies, his 1832 paper was the first written on the subject. Ironically, Hodgkin's pioneering study, made when microscopic examination of tissues was virtually unknown, went unrecognized for twenty-four years. Dr. Samuel Wilks rediscovered Hodgkin's manuscript in 1856 and wrote another treatise on the disorder, adding his own observations. Then, in what may be the greatest act of magnanimity recorded in the whole history of medicine, Wilks named the malady Hodgkin's disease rather than having it named after himself. Ninety-seven years after Hodgkin's original work, tissues from the first three cases, preserved in spirits, were examined microscopically, and the diagnosis was confirmed.

In spite of his brilliance, Hodgkin managed to suffer some discrimination because of his Quaker dress and his considerable eccentricities. Devoting much time to philanthropic activities, he was careless in collecting fees and never had a large practice. Hodgkin died tragically of dysentery in Jaffa during a visit to Palestine in the middle of a cholera epidemic, while he was attempting to relieve the miseries of Jews in the Middle East. Hodgkin's disease comprises 40 percent of a group of disorders called the lymphomas, all characterized by a malignant overgrowth of the cells of the lymphatic system. Lymphatic tissue is found, not only in the chains of lymph nodes throughout the body, but also in the spleen and bowel, and ordinarily plays a role in immunity and defense against disease. About 50 percent of all Hodgkin's disease occurs between the ages of twenty and forty, with less than 10 percent either after age sixty or before age ten. Males are affected 33 percent more often than females and tend to fare worse than their women counterparts.

What causes Hodgkin's disease? In spite of exhaustive research, no single agent has been uncovered. For over a century an infectious organism—a bacteria or virus—has been sought because the chills and fever seen in the later stages are so suggestive of infection, and because the tissue changes are so similar to those of tuberculosis. The identification of viruslike agents in cultures of tissue taken from Hodgkins disease patients, as well as other evidence, has strongly suggested to many researchers that a virus must be involved. In addition, studies of the distribution of the malady have revealed an increased incidence in certain groups with moderately close contact. Of course, serious social consequences could ensue from labeling Hodgkin's patients infectious, so much stronger evidence must be obtained before this is done.

The disease is usually first noticed when painless lumps—enlarged lymph nodes—appear in one side of the neck. Later, nodes in the armpit, the groin, or the opposite side of the neck may also enlarge. Fever, sweating, weight loss, and generalized itching are other frequent complaints.

Because of the obvious signs, diagnosis of Hodgkin's disease is not difficult to make in most cases. If an enlarged lymph node is present in the neck, the node can be removed through a small skin incision and examined microscopically. Besides the distortion of the normal cellular structure by tumor, a special malignant cell, the so-called Reed Sternberg cell, is present in the cancerous tissue of all Hodgkin's patients.

Once the diagnosis has been made, the chance of surviving five years can be ascertained by examining two factors: (1) the stage of the disease, and (2) the type of cells found.

Staging   Stage I disease has involved only a single chain of lymph nodes, for example, in one side of the neck, or two contiguous nodal chains.

Stage II disease affects two or more noncontiguous groups of lymph nodes, but these are on the same side of the diaphragm. An example would be diseased chains of lymph nodes on both sides of the neck.

Stage III disease involves lymph node chains on both sides of the diaphragm, or an extralymphatic organ such as liver or spleen. Enlarged lymph nodes in both the neck and the groin would indicate stage III disease.

Stage IV disease is diffuse or disseminated Hodgkin's disease involving such organs as bone, skin, or bone marrow. Lymph nodes may or may not be enlarged.

Each stage, in addition, is divided into categories A and B, B for patients with certain general symptoms and A for those without. Symptoms are: (1) unexplained weight loss of more than 10 percent of body weight in the previous six months, (2) unexplained fevers, and (3) night sweats.

Cell Type   In the Lukes classification of Hodgkin cells, now the most generally accepted, there are four cell types, which can be recognized microscopically:

Lymphocyte predominant, making up 5 percent of cases, confers the best outlook.

Nodular sclerosis comprises 52 percent of cases and is slightly less favorable than lymphocyte predominant.

Mixed cellularity accounts for 3 percent of cases and is less favorable than nodular sclerosis.

Lymphocyte depleted, making up only 6 percent of cases, has the worst outlook. Few of these patients will survive their disease in spite of the most vigorous therapeutic measures.

Treatment   Besides being important in determining outlook, knowledge of the stage of the disease is also vital in prescribing treatment. For this reason, an effort to determine stage is made immediately after confirmation of the diagnosis. Since some lymph nodes within the abdominal cavity cannot be inspected visually or palpated, a special X-ray procedure, lymphangiography, is employed. This requires the injection of an oily compound through a very fine needle into one of the small lymphatic vessels within a toe web. The oil is taken up by the lymph nodes in the abdomen, then visualized on X-ray films. In order to stage even more exactly, physicians open the abdomen surgically to remove the spleen, inspect lymph nodes, and take a small piece of liver tissue. Although doctors once believed that patients without a spleen fared better after treatment, there is now not so much certainty of this.

Radiation therapy is the primary form of treatment for all stages of Hodgkin's disease, save the disseminated stage IV. Cobalt sixty and other sources of high-energy X ray have substantially increased the cure rate of this once hopeless malady. From Stanford University Hospital, Dr. Henry Kaplan and his associates report an 89 percent five-year survival for those stage I cases with lymphocyte predominant cell type.

The method of radiating the patient is known as segmental sequential irradiation or, more commonly, total nodal irradiation. Because Hodgkin's disease appears to begin in a single group of nodes and then spread successively to adjacent node groups, a whole block of such groups, rather than a single group, is treated at once. Above the diaphragm this block is referred to as a mantle because it is shaped to encompass all chest nodes, neck nodes, and nodes in the armpits. Below the diaphragm the radiated area takes the form of an inverted Y in order for the X rays to hit the abdominal nodes lying in a chain along the spine and the nodes in the groin. During treatment great care is taken to shield such vital structures as the lungs and the kidneys from the X-ray beam.

In the advanced stages of Hodgkin's disease, stages III and IV, chemotherapy (drug treatment) has recently entered an exciting new era in which long-term complete remissions and apparent disease-free periods can be effected in over half of previously untreated patients. Even in stage I and II cases, where radiation is still the mainstay of therapy, chemotherapy is now being administered in some cases where early spread of disease is suspected. A combination of nitrogen mustard, vincristine (Oncovin), procarbazine, and prednisone has been found especially effective; this is called the "MOPP" regimen for short.

Hodgkin's disease during pregnancy merits special consideration. Therapeutic abortion does not, in general, seem warranted, since the malady is not accelerated in a pregnant woman; however, females with active disease are advised against becoming pregnant because their survival outlook is so uncertain. Doctors usually tell such patients to wait until the disease has been in remission for two years, as the majority of relapses occur during this period. During pregnancy itself no treatment is given.

The outlook and length of survival after treatment can be correlated with the stage and cell type of the disease when diagnosed, as has been mentioned. But the appearance of such symptoms as fever or itching, and the involvement of bone or liver by malignant cells, considerably reduce the chance for recovery. Some representative figures reported by two institutions are shown in Table 1.

Non-Hodgkin's Lymphoma

This group of disorders, including reticulum cell sarcoma, lymphosarcoma, giant follicular lymphoma, and others, usually occurs in an older age group than does Hodgkin's disease. Men

Table 1

Survival Rate of Hodgkins Disease Patients
after Treatment

Physician and Institution	Stage	Survival 5 year	10 year
Dr. Vera Peters	I	67%	46%
Princess Margaret Hospital	II	55%	31%
Toronto, Canada (1931–65)	III	23%	8%
	IV	9%	1%
Dr. Henry Kaplan	I	89%	
Stanford University	II	67%	
Medical Center	III	42%	
Stanford, California (1972)	IV	20%	

predominate over women 1.7 to 1; incidence peaks between the ages of sixty and sixty-nine. Hodgkin's disease is more than twice as common as any malignancy in this category.

As in Hodgkin's disease, a causative virus has been incriminated in at least a few of the non-Hodgkin's lymphomas. Some of the evidence, drawn from studies of Burkitt's lymphoma (see chapter 1), electron microscopy, and cell culture, seems to implicate a herpeslike virus. (Herpes simplex virus is known to cause "cold sores.") Further suggestions of a viral culprit were reported by Dr. I. Penn in 1972, in the journal *Transplantation*. Patients receiving kidney transplants are given special drugs called immunosuppresssives to prevent rejection of the new organ by inactivating normal rejection mechanisms. These same mechanisms also normally fight viral infections. An unusual form of reticulum cell sarcoma was found to appear with abnormally high frequency in these individuals.

Symptoms and signs in patients with non-Hodgkin's lymphomas are similar to those of Hodgkin's disease; the diseases often can only be distinguished by microscopic examination of a cancer tissue specimen. A representative case is that of Charles Lindbergh.

In 1972, a surgeon performing a routine preoperative examination on Lindbergh found an abnormal lymph node that proved to contain lymphoma. Since another node above the collarbone was also noted to be involved, the poor outlook was promptly and honestly reported to the patient himself. Radiation therapy produced a welcome remission for a time, and Lindbergh was able to travel extensively on his many conservation missions. These included the preservation of a rare species of eagle and the study of the Stone Age Tasaday tribe in the Philippines. Chemotherapy with multiple drugs was also instituted and carried to the limit of its effectiveness.

From time to time, the famed aviator managed to return to Kipahulu Valley, on the island of Maui, Hawaii, a living museum of tropical foliage and wildlife. His contributions of time and effort had been considerable in preserving the area as a national park. Near this valley of a thousand waterfalls, Lindbergh had personally helped clear the neglected graveyard beside the small church built by Yankee missionaries, and it was this spot that he selected for the site of his burial.

In 1974, Lindbergh's deteriorating condition forced his hospitalization in the Columbia Presbyterian Medical Center, New York City. By August, the flier knew he had only a few days left. He called the village of Hana, Hawaii, from his hospital room. "This is Charles Lindbergh. I have had a conference with my doctors, and they advise me that I have only a short time to live. Please find me a cottage or cabin near the village. I am coming home to Maui."

Because of his great wealth—his wife Anne Morrow Lindbergh is the daughter of Dwight Morrow, a former Morgan banking partner—Lindbergh was able to fly to Hawaii with his physician, two nurses, and his family. Here he passed the last eight days of his life.

The first few days brought elation; appetite improved, and fluid intake as well. The dying man had regular morning conferences with his ranch superintendent to give instructions and receive reports on the construction of his tomb and the building of his coffin. When his lungs filled with fluid, oxygen was administered, as well as codeine for pain. Finally coma supervened, with death coming twelve hours later. Lindbergh wisely refused all life-sustaining measures. As in Hodgkin's disease, radiation therapy is the mainstay of treatment in non-Hodgkin's lymphoma. Chemotherapy is much less effective, and fewer remissions or apparent disease-free periods can be produced with drugs. Although patients with giant follicular lymphoma may live quite a long time, the overall survival for non-Hodgkin's lymphoma patients is considerably lower than in Hodgkin's disease, as is illustrated by Charles Lindberg's case. There has, however, been some increased survival in the past twenty-five years due to higher radiation doses over more extended areas.

Multiple Myeloma

Multiple myeloma is a cancer caused by a malignant overgrowth of a special cell within the bone marrow, the plasma cell. Its normal function is to produce blood proteins called globulins that provide immunity. The cancerous plasma cells form large amounts of an abnormal globulin, Bence-Jones protein, that can be detected in blood and urine. The homogeneous nature of this compound suggests that malignant transformation of a single cell or small group of cells is responsible for the disorder. Viruslike particles have been observed with the electron microscope in both human and mouse plasma cell tumors, but the reason for the presence of virus remains obscure.

Though no causative organism has been identified, sex and age play a role. Men are more commonly affected than women by multiple myeloma, and most patients are between fifty and seventy years of age. About nine persons in every million can be expected to develop the disorder, making it one of the rarer forms of cancer.

The disease is commonly discovered after patients see their physician complaining of back pain and laboratory tests reveal anemia. A typical case was that of Frank McGee, the host of

NBC's "Today" program. In spite of the severe bone pain, McGee was able to continue working until shortly before his death, when he was literally quivering with pain and unable even to sit. Reluctant to discuss with colleagues the real nature of his illness, he continually insisted that he had only a bad back, though everyone knew that something worse must have been responsible for the unrelenting agony. Multiple hospitalizations and treatment with drugs and radiotherapy did provide some relief, and while in the hospital McGee was able to retain his charming television personality, waving and chatting amiably, acknowledging with pleasure his recognition by other patients. When last seen by his radiation therapist during his final hospitalization, McGee was reading *Alive,* the story of the ordeal of soccer players whose plane crashed in the Andes, and he volunteered to lend the book to the doctor in two days when he was through. "And I promise it won't be tear stained," he added with a smile. Asked how sitting so long before a television camera was possible in his condition, he revealed that the secret was simply not to move. A few days later, McGee died of an overwhelming pneumonia only a few blocks uptown from the NBC studios in New York City, where so much of his career had been spent.

As in the case of Frank McGee, chemotherapy, especially with the drugs cytoxan and melphalan, can produce great relief from the symptoms of multiple myeloma. Radiation therapy is also of value in relieving pain from specific local lesions and in healing fractured, diseased bones. Blood transfusions are frequently given to reduce the degree of anemia. But this disease is incurable, and most afflicted individuals will die within two years.

Waldenstrom's Macroglobulinemia

This uncommon condition, seen most often in men over fifty, causes symptoms similar to those of a slowly progressive lymphoma. An abnormal viscous blood protein called a macroglobulin is produced by malignant cells similar to plasma cells;

many normal functions are gummed up by the compound's sluggish presence. Bleeding tendencies may be prominent, probably because of improper clotting. Visual disturbances result from impaired retinal circulation secondary to increased blood viscosity. Fatigue and weight loss, anemia, lymph node enlargement, and heart failure are also part of the total picture.

9 Tumors of the Nervous System

Tumors of the central nervous sysem—the brain and spinal cord—are not rare. In a 1958 study, the statistician L. T. Kurland estimated that about fifteen thousand new primary brain tumors and four thousand new spinal cord tumors occurred each year, and these accounted for 2 percent of all cancer deaths. When these figures are combined with the number of metastatic tumors to the central nervous system, that is, with cancers that begin in other places such as the lung, the total is two to five times as great. An especially famous case was that of one of America's most gifted musical composers.

On the evening of February 11, 1937, an enthusiastic Los Angeles audience applauded the performance of George Gershwin. The event was the second in a series of all-Gershwin programs that the musician had agreed to perform with the Los Angeles Philharmonic while living temporarily in Hollywood. Unknown to most of the audience, however, was the fact that, while playing his Concerto in F, Gershwin had experienced a momentary blackout. The conductor, Alexander Smallens, expertly disguised the brief interruption until his guest artist recovered and rejoined the orchestra several bars later. This was the first evidence of failing coordination, which heralded Gershwin's tragic and untimely death several months later.

The youthful American composer had rapidly risen to fame in Tin Pan Alley with his catchy tunes and soon achieved phenomenal success as a creator of Broadway musicals. Then he turned to more serious pursuits, and his *Rhapsody in Blue* and *Concerto in F* were recognized by musical critics as revolutionary compositions. In 1933 he completed the opera *Porgy and Bess,* perhaps the greatest achievement of his career. Gershwin experienced several more brief episodes of unconsciousness during the spring of 1937, and each was preceded by the sensation of "smelling burning rubber." Complaints such as these came as no surprise to family and friends, since Gershwin had suffered for years from innumerable symptoms that could not satisfactorily be explained by his doctors. Chronic constipation and persistent gastric distress led him to include large quantities of agar, rusk, and melba toast in his diet. "Nobody believes me when I say I'm sick," he would carp endlessly.

Prior to the appearance of blackout spells, George and his brother-lyricist Ira had been working feverishly for nearly twelve months on the score of *Shall We Dance,* a musical film extravaganza starring Fred Astaire and Ginger Rogers. Most of Gershwin's friends attributed his increasing physical complaints to the strain of working in Hollywood and urged him to return to New York. But he refused.

The composer had been in psychoanalysis for several years; now, with an increase in frequency of headaches and dizziness, his psychiatrist recommended a complete neurological evaluation. Gershwin entered Cedars of Lebanon Hospital early in June, the sense of smelling strange odors remaining his only noteworthy symptom. One useful diagnostic procedure in these cases is a spinal tap, the insertion of a long, hollow needle into the spinal canal to withdraw a sample of spinal fluid. Since this procedure was adamantly rejected, further diagnostic efforts were terminated, and the patient was discharged.

At home, Gershwin slept for longer and longer periods each day, until finally he could not get up at all, much less play the piano. On the morning of July 9, he passed into a semicomatose state; he was rushed back to Cedars of Lebanon later that afternoon. Dr. Carl Rand, a neurosurgeon, was summoned and immediately performed a spinal tap that revealed marked abnormalities.

Meanwhile Dr. Howard Naffziger of the University of California Medical Center in San Francisco and Dr. Walter Dandy, the famed Johns Hopkins neurosurgeon, had been called. Upon arrival the next day, Dr. Naffziger recognized the immediate need for surgery. Dandy was stopped at the Newark, New Jersey, airport with the news that Naffziger had decided to proceed with the operation.

At surgery, a large tumor was found in the left side of the brain, and only partial removal was possible. Gershwin never regained consciousness and died the next day, July 11, 1937. Subsequent microscopic examination revealed a highly malignant lesion. After receiving the final report, Dr. Dandy wrote a brief note to Dr. Naffziger stating that, in his experience, very few such growths were curable. Surgery might have prolonged life slightly, but the almost inevitable recurrence would surely have produced a slow, insidious death, a difficult experience for such a brilliant and creative person.

George Gershwin's brain tumor was a glioma, a type that makes up the majority of central nervous system malignancies. Although rarely spreading beyond the central nervous system, all gliomas are considered malignant because they invade the surrounding brain tissue, and complete removal is usually not possible. Despite advances in neurosurgery and radiotherapy, central nervous system tumors are still associated with a high degree of complications and mortality. The predisposition to remain contained within the skull and spinal canal would suggest that radiation could offer a successful means of control, but alas, the radiation doses required may irreparably damage the normal tissue as well; even patients who survive can develop seizures or other late effects. But adding drug therapy to surgery and radiation is sometimes effective for one childhood tumor, medulloblastoma, and the combination is being actively investigated for tumors of adults.

The most common adult tumor, the glioma, can be highly

malignant and fast growing, or slow growing and occasionally curable. Most often the onset is between the ages of forty and sixty. Glioblastoma multiforme is another name given to the most malignant glioma, while astrocytoma is used interchangeably with glioma. Astrocytomas are graded from I to IV, with grade III or IV being synonymous with glioblastoma multiforme. Survival ranges from several years with the low-grade tumors to less than a year in the case of glioblastoma multiforme. A rare form of glioma, the ependymoma, is highly malignant when found in the brain but may be very slow growing if originating in the spinal cord.

Meningioma is the most common of the nongliomatous adult tumors and develops from the meninges, a thin layer of connective tissue that lines the skull and spinal canal. Usually slow growing, these lesions can often be completely removed to achieve a cure. Sometimes only a partial excision is possible, but even so there will be great symptomatic relief with recurrence a problem only after many years.

When the pituitary gland, the controller of the other endocrine glands, develops a tumor, some of the symptoms may be hormonal. One such tumor, the basophilic adenoma, secretes a substance that stimulates the adrenal glands to produce an excess of the hormone cortisol, leading in turn to a moon face, a buffalo-humped back, stretch marks on the skin, poor wound healing, and demineralization of the bones. This set of manifestations is called Cushing's disease after Dr. Harvey Cushing, the gifted Harvard neurosurgeon who first described it. Among Cushing's other accomplishments was the fathering of three distinguished daughters: Mrs. William Paley (formerly Mrs. Stanley G. Mortimer), second wife of the board chairman of CBS and chosen by the New York Dress Institute in 1945 as best-dressed woman in the world; Mrs. John Hay Whitney, wife of the former publisher of the New York *Herald Tribune*; and Mrs. Vincent Astor.

A second pituitary tumor, the acidophilic adenoma, leads to the production of excess growth hormone. If the condition appears before puberty, a giant is the result. After puberty, a disease called acromegaly emerges: patients develop enlargement of hands and feet, a jutting lower jaw, and soft tissue and bony changes in the face.

Nonfunctioning pituitary tumors—those growths that cause no hormone overproduction—lead to three types of symptoms and signs, all from pressure. Headache is common. Partial blindness occurs after a part of the optic nerve is affected. And diabetes insipidus, the overexcretion of urine without sugar abnormalities, results from destruction of the section of pituitary known as the neurohypophysis; this part of the gland normally produces antidiuretic hormone, a protein that regulates kidney function. Solid nonfunctioning tumors are usually chromophobe adenomas, but craniopharyngioma, a cystic tumor, and dermoid, another solid tumor, can also be found.

Children may be afflicted with a special brain tumor, the medulloblastoma. This lesion develops within the cerebellum, a part of the brain at the posterior base of the skull very close to the brain stem. Normally, all of the voluntary muscles instantaneously telegraph their positions and states of contraction to the cerebellum so that physical actions, including speech and eye movement, may be precisely coordinated. But as the rapidly growing cells of the medulloblastoma proceed to destroy the cerebellum, coordination is lost. The child becomes clumsy, trips, and speaks in a garbled manner.

Tumors of the spinal cord are similar to those of the brain. Two-thirds of these tumors are nonmalignant—either meningiomas or neurofibromas (which develop from nerve sheaths). All spinal cord growths, however, are much less frequent than their counterparts in the brain and are quite rare in childhood and old age. The first symptoms are usually pain and tingling in a limb followed by sensory loss, muscular weakness, and wasting. Growth of the tumor leads to spinal cord compression, spastic weakness, and impaired skin sensation in localized regions. A very low tumor may affect voluntary control of the bladder and bowel.

Making a positive diagnosis of a tumor of the brain was once a complicated process. Skull X rays, spinal tap, electroencephalogram, and radioisotopic brain scan were de rigueur. But most feared were two rather formidable X-ray studies, the cerebral angiogram and the pneumoencephalogram. The angiogram requires injection under pressure of an iodine-containing liquid into the neck artery in order to fill the vessels of the brain and make them visible on an X ray. The pneumoencephalogram, devised by Johns Hopkins's Dr. Walter Dandy in 1918, necessitates removing fluid via a spinal tap and injecting air—an excruciatingly painful maneuver—for X-ray visualization of the cavities within the interior of the brain. Frightful complications can occur after both these techniques, causing death or permanent disability in some patients. Fortunately, a brilliant invention announced in 1972 has made the pneumoencephalogram practically obsolete, and has reduced the need for cerebral angiography.

A British engineer, Dr. Godfrey Hounsfield, employing a numerical technique developed by an Austrian mathematician, A. Radon, in 1917, constructed the first computerized axial tomographic (CAT) scanner. This ingenious device uses X rays and a computer to reconstruct cross-sectional images of the brain and body as simply and harmlessly as a routine chest X ray.

Diagnosis of spinal cord tumors has traditionally also been effected with an X-ray study, myelography. A thick, iodine-containing oil is introduced through a spinal tap, with X rays then used to demonstrate the lesion outlined by the column of oil within the spinal canal. Recently, though, CAT scanners have proven to be a great help in identifying spinal tumors, as well as differentiating them from other conditions. In the future, perhaps, myelography may become as obsolete as pneumoencephalography.

The initial treatment of almost all primary brain and spinal cord tumors is surgical exploration. As with tumors elsewhere in the body, removal is limited by the malignancy and invasiveness of the growth in question. In addition, technical problems and inaccessibility at the time of operation may make removal of even a benign lesion impossible. As has been mentioned, meningiomas can often be completely excised; so can neurofibromas. Regrettably, however, astrocytomas and other malignant brain and spinal cord tumors can be cured only rarely. Generally, by the time of discovery, invasion of deep-seated areas of the brain has already occurred, preventing complete extirpation. In such cases, the surgeon usually attempts to remove as much of the tumor as possible, relieving pressure and restoring function temporarily.

Most malignant brain tumors respond to radiation therapy, even those not partially taken out. A course of such treatment generally adds to the patient's longevity and at times will even allay symptoms when tumors recur. Radiation can actually cure a large percentage of medulloblastomas in children, but malignant brain tumors in general appear to become less sensitive to X rays as patients age. Only rarely is surgery performed when a brain tumor is known to be metastatic from another organ; radiation is the principal mode of therapy here. But benign tumors such as meningiomas and neurofibromas are very resistant to even the highest radiation doses; surgery is employed almost exclusively in these cases.

Chemotherapy with various drugs is being actively investigated for all forms of brain tumors. Although no firm evidence of benefit has yet emerged, results are promising, particularly with medulloblastomas and glioblastoma multiforme. The drug methotrexate appears especially valuable in such cases. Cortisone, the antiinflammatory adrenal gland hormone, is administered to most patients to decrease the swelling of the brain that almost inevitably accompanies malignant tumors.

How would George Gershwin have fared if treated today? More than likely the combination of cortisone and high-energy radiation therapy, both unavailable in 1937, would have allowed him to regain consciousness and live for a few months. But his chances of long-term survival still would be quite slim.

10 Tumors of the Eye

Two main kinds of malignant tumors develop within the eye: retinoblastoma, a tumor of children (see chapter 13); and malignant melanoma.

Malignant melanoma? Isn't that a skin tumor? Unfortunately, malignant melanomas have the lamentable habit of turning up in sites other than the skin. The eye is a bad location because of the therapy involved.

Of the malignant tumors that grow within the eye, malignant melanoma is the most common, though it makes up a relatively small portion of all melanomas. The peak incidence is between fifty and sixty years of age, with no predisposition for male or female, though blacks are rarely affected.

Many melanomas begin in the choroid, a thin, vessel-filled layer of tissue that lies behind and nourishes the light-sensitive retina. As the tumor grows, it can produce a retinal detachment, stripping away the retina from the wall of the eye. Patients get a sudden sensation of a curtain obscuring vision, then grow blind in the affected eye. Visual impairment will occur much earlier should the growth begin behind the section of retina known as the macula lutea, the most vital portion for clear vision. Glaucoma, an elevation of fluid pressure within the eye, can occur if the tumor blocks the avenues of fluid outflow. Some melanomas begin from pigmented moles on the iris.

If melanoma is detected as a small lesion on the iris, the tumor itself can be excised and the eye saved; the only treatment for other forms of intraocular melanoma is removal of the eye—enucleation. So accurate diagnosis is of utmost importance, and elaborate methods have been tried, such as injecting the dye fluorescein into the retinal arteries, or studying lesions with the radioactive isotope phosphorus-32. Removal of a tissue sample for microscopic examination is not possible because of the spread of tumor that occurs after the deep perforation of the eye with a needle. Most commonly an ophthalmologist uses an optical instrument, the ophthalmoscope, to look through the pupil and visualize the lesion. But diagnostic accuracy is only fair. A 1964 study of 744 cases of eyes enucleated for melanoma revealed errors in 100 cases. Hemorrhage, ordinary retinal detachment, retinal cysts, and other conditions were responsible for the mistakes.

The size of an intraocular melanoma has a direct bearing on the outlook for survival; larger tumors are associated with higher mortality. The results of enucleation are good if the tumor is small and has not extended outside of the eye. But the ordinary five-year survival rate is not an adequate measure of cure, because distant lesions may develop ten to fifteen years after the eye has been removed. Evidently the metastatic tumor cells may lie dormant for many years; what excites their eventual growth is unknown.

As vulnerable to cancer as the eye itself are the supporting structures around the eye. Most commonly affected are the eyelids, which are susceptible to skin cancers of the basal and squamous cell variety (see chapter 7). Typically such lesions present as a sore that fails to heal or a persistent warty growth. Definitive diagnosis is made by removing a small piece of the tumor for microscopic examination. If treatment is surgical, a wide excision must be made to remove all tumor cells. Radiation therapy, on the other hand, creates no defect or scar, but will cause the lashes to be lost. This may be a significant cosmetic blemish on the upper lid, but is much less so for the lower lid, where most cancers occur. Postirradiation bleaching and shrinking of the tissues may also produce an undesirable appearance after radiotherapy.

11 Tumors of the Head and Neck

To the cancer specialist, head and neck tumors include those found in the oral cavity, the nose and paranasal sinuses, the larynx, and the salivary glands. This group of lesions produces some of the most acrimonious debate between surgeons and radiotherapists, because surgery and radiation are competitive and of roughly comparable value in producing cure. But these treatment methods are also often mutually exclusive; a patient receiving therapy extensive enough to be cured by one technique can hardly ever be successfully retreated by the other should the tumor recur. Surgeons have a tactical advantage in most hospitals because the cases are initially referred to them for treatment. A radiotherapist will usually get a case for one of three reasons: (1) the patient refuses the surgery because of the cosmetic and functional impairment, (2) the tumor recurs after surgery and the patient is sent for radiation for lack of other alternatives, or (3) the tumor is too extensive for surgery.

The Tongue

Malignant tumors of the oral cavity make up about 5 percent of all cancer occurring in the human body. These tumors have a distinct character and survival outlook, depending upon point of origin. The tongue itself demonstrates the whole survival spectrum, with small lesions on the tip having a very good outlook after proper treatment, while for posterior lesions the prognosis is dismal. Recent studies have delineated the predominant cause for this form of cancer: the combination of immoderate drinking and smoking, though an excess of either may be enough. A perfect example of a typical case can be found in the life of Ulysses S. Grant.

Grant first began to smoke and drink heavily while serving as an army officer. After years of exposure to cigars and whiskey, a carcinoma developed at the base of his tongue. At the time, Grant was writing his memoirs for publication, since he had gone bankrupt after some ill-advised financial speculation. In the nineteenth century, there was no treatment for a lesion such as Grant had, and so the finishing of the memoirs became a race with death. He completed the last chapter only a week before he died. Mark Twain, the publisher, sold three hundred thousand copies of the work; the royalties provided more than $450,000 to Grant's widow.

A base-of-tongue cancer such as Grant's has a better outlook now than it had in the 1880s, but not much better. Because this region is so richly supplied with blood and lymphatic vessels, the tumor tends to spread early and rapidly. Radiation therapy is an effective means of treatment. Surgery is also effective but may be more disabling because a portion of the tongue is removed. After adequate treatment, 20 percent of patients can be expected to survive five years.

The big dispute between surgeons and radiotherapists occurs over lesions in the mid-portion or tip of the tongue. Surgery and radiation are of roughly comparable effectiveness, but after an operation there is inevitable disfigurement and loss of function. Speech will be slurred, swallowing is incomplete, saliva is drooled constantly, and even a cured patient will have large, ugly scars. Radiation therapy, on the other hand, will produce none of these distressing sequelae in most cases. Unfortunately, many patients are not aware of the differences between the two forms of therapy, and so curative radiation is not applied as often as its effectiveness warrants.

A problem in the treatment of all oral cancers is the predisposition for recurrence at a nearby site. Patients who have been successfully treated will almost invariably continue to smoke, or to smoke and drink, if such is their pleasure. Stern warnings and the disfigurement of the first operation almost never discourage continued exposure to smoke and alcohol, and death finally comes as a result of a second or even third cancer. A famous case of palate cancer illustrates this fact.

The Palate

Like Ulysses S. Grant, Sigmund Freud was a heavy smoker, consuming as many as twenty cigars per day. Psychiatrists claim that one of the major reasons for smoking is oral gratification, an unconscious return to the mother's breast. But Freud once poked some fun at this notion, holding up a long black cigar before a group of his students and saying, "Just remember, it is not always a symbol—sometimes it's just a cigar." Freud also had the habit of hawking and spitting due to a chronic nasal and sinus infection, which was undoubtedly aggravated by the excessive smoking. Patients unaccustomed to such behavior were disturbed by it, whereupon Freud chided them for their squeamishness. Freud's efforts to reduce or abolish his smoking were ineffective. During one fourteen-month period of abstinence, he described the effects: "Soon after giving up smoking, there were intolerable days. . . . Then there came suddenly a severe affliction of the heart, worse than I ever had when smoking. The maddest racing and irregularity, constant cardiac tension, oppression, burning, hot pain down the left arm, some dyspnea of a suspiciously organic degree—all that in two or three attacks a day and continuing. And with it an oppression of mood in which images of dying and farewell scenes replaced the more usual fantasies about one's occupation." And so the smoking continued.

Shortly before his sixty-seventh birthday, Freud noticed the first evidence of oral cancer, a whitish, premalignant change called leukoplakia. He did nothing about it for two months, making no mention of his suspicions to anyone. In a letter written in English to his biographer, Dr. Ernest Jones, on April

25, 1923, Freud declared, "I detected two months ago a leu-koplastic growth on my jaw and palate right side which I had removed on the twentieth. I am still out of work and cannot swallow. I was assured of the benignity of the matter but as you know, nobody can guarantee its behavior when it be permitted to grow further. My own diagnosis had been epithelioma, but was not accepted. Smoking is accused as the etiology of this tissue rebellion."

Several days before writing this letter, Freud had consulted Dr. Marcus Hajek, a Viennese nose and throat specialist and an old acquaintance. In reply to a question asked by Freud, Hajek cooly made the ominous remark, "No one can be expected to live forever." Hajek advised removal of the growth, called the procedure trivial, and declared that the excision could readily be performed in his outpatient clinic. Previously a dermatologist also had examined Freud, making a diagnosis of leukoplakia and advising excision. Ernest Jones relates what happened subsequently.

> After a few days of reflection Freud quietly turned up at Hajek's clinic without saying a word to anyone at home. . . . Presently the family were surprised by getting a tele-phone message from the clinic requesting them to bring a few necessities for him to stay the night. Wife and daughter hurried there to find Freud sitting on a kitchen chair in the outpatient department with blood all over his clothes. The operation had not gone as had been expected, and the loss of blood had been so considerable that it was not advisable for the patient to return home. There was no free room or even a bed in the clinic, but a bed was rigged up in a small room. . . . The ward sister sent the two ladies home at lunch time . . . and assured them the patient would be all right. . . . When they returned an hour or two later they learned that he had an attack of pro-fuse bleeding. . . . After some difficulty the bleeding was stopped. . . . Anna Freud then refused to leave again and spent the night sitting by her father's side. He was weak from loss of blood, was half drugged from the medicines,

and was in great pain. . . . The next morning Hajek demonstrated the case to a crowd of students, and later in the
day Freud was allowed to go home. So ended the first of
thirty-three operations Freud underwent before he ultimately found release.

Freud saw Hajek several times during the next few months,
and the surgeon raised no objection to Freud's going away for
his customary three months' holiday, but startled Freud when
he asked him to send a report of his condition every two weeks
and to appear personally at the end of July. When in mid-July
Freud wrote to inquire whether he really need come, Hajek,
after a delay, answered that it wasn't necessary and that he
could stay away the entire summer. This ambiguity made Freud
increasingly distrustful of the surgeon.

So Freud asked his physician, Dr. Felix Deutsch, for an
examination. Deutsch found a recurrence of the growth. Dr.
Hans Pichler, a distinguished oral surgeon, was called in con-
sultation, and on September 26, 1923, he and Hajek found an
unmistakable malignant ulcer on the hard palate, with cancerous invasion of the neighboring tissues including the upper
part of the lower jaw and the cheek. On October 4 and 11,
Pichler operated in two stages. During the first operation, the
external carotid artery in the neck was ligated and the sub-
maxillary salivary glands—some of which were suspiciously enlarged—removed. In the second operation, the surgeon removed "the whole upper jaw and palate on the affected side, a
very extensive operation which threw the nasal cavity and
mouth into one." As both operations were performed under
local anesthesia, Freud's tolerance for pain must have been
indeed prodigious.

To shut off the mouth from the nasal cavity and make speech
and eating possible, a huge, ungainly prosthesis was designed,
which was labeled "the monster." So difficult was the removal
and replacement of this cumbersome device that, on one occa-
sion, the combined efforts of Freud and his daughter failed to
insert it after a half-hour struggle; the surgeon had to be called

for this purpose. The tight fit necessary to make speaking and eating possible produced constant, intolerable irritation. But if the device was left out for more than a few hours, the tissues would shrink, and reintroduction was not feasible unless the prosthesis was physically altered.

As could be expected, the large surgical defect and the prosthesis caused an abnormality in Freud's speech. Its quality became nasal and thick, rather like that of someone with a cleft palate. Eating also became a trial seldom performed in company. Hearing impairment from constant infections led to almost total deafness on the right side, forcing a change in position of Freud's chair and psychoanalytic couch so that patients could still be heard.

On November 12, 1923, a third operation was performed. Five days later Freud had a vasectomy at his own request because, he said, altered hormone production might inhibit the growth of the cancer. More likely, the combination of the cancer and the vascular disease produced by years of smoking had rendered Freud impotent—certainly no surprise in a sixty-seven-year-old man. Vasectomy, then called the Steinach operation, was erroneously believed to help restore potency; perhaps this rejuvenation was what the great psychiatrist really hoped for.

For the last sixteen years of his life, Freud was forced to endure endless discomfort, pain, and treatment with X rays, radium, and diathermy. An attack of influenza in March, 1924, left disagreeable nasal and sinus aftereffects. Endless problems with the prosthesis meant modifications every few days. In February, a second prosthesis was made, and in October still a third, lamentably with little relief. In order to get a cigar between his teeth, Freud had to force his bite open with the assistance of a clothes peg. This situation suggests that of a heavy smoker who has lost his larynx from cancer and his hands from vascular disease, all secondary to tobacco; he manages to continue smoking by grasping the cigarette in his metal claw and inhaling through the tracheostomy orifice in the middle of his neck.

Because of the endless struggle to improve the prosthesis, a number of minor operations were performed in June, 1925. A fourth prosthesis, made the following year, like the others failed to relieve discomfort. Freud wrote to a fellow analyst in August, 1927, of "being eternally ill and plagued with discomfort." By the spring of 1928, when the discomfort and pain in Freud's mouth had become almost unbearable, a famous Berlin oral surgeon was summoned to make another prosthesis. The new device, though imperfect, proved to be better than the previous ones, and life became more tolerable, at least until May, 1930, when another prosthesis had to be made.

In Febuary, 1931, "another suspicious spot" was dealt with by electrocoagulation, and in April, a large section of tissue was excised. Dr. Jacob Erdheim, an outstanding Viennese pathologist, examined the precancerous tissue and concluded that nicotine was the causative agent. Again Freud refused to renounce smoking, maintaining that abstinence from tobacco was not justified at his age.

Severe influenza, a middle-ear infection that lasted more than a month, and five operations filled the year 1932. By 1934 X-ray and radium treatments were employed extensively. In July, 1936, Freud underwent two painful operations, and for the first time since the original operation in 1923, unmistakable cancer was detected. Late in the year another suspicious area was removed, and it was during this procedure that Freud cried, "I can't go on any longer."

On March 11, 1938, the Nazis annexed Austria. Several influential friends were able to arrange for Freud and his family to leave for England the following spring. In September the longest operation was performed—two and a quarter hours. Freud wrote that this was the most severe surgery he had ever had, and he was left frightfully weak and practically unable to write or talk.

The last two years of life were the worst. Suspicious areas no longer proved to be precancerous, but were definitely malignant. In February a swelling occurred, gradually taking on an ominous look that was finally labeled "inoperable, incurable cancer." As Freud's condition began to deteriorate, loss of weight and signs of apathy appeared. Ulcerations formed as the tumor invaded the cheek, causing the wound to emit a noxious odor. When a radio broadcast announced that World War II was to be the last war, one of his physicians asked Freud whether he believed this. "Anyhow it is my last war," was the reply. A few days later, on September 23, 1939, death came to the father of psychoanalysis.

This case graphically illustrates the difficulties involved in treating the oral cancer of a smoker. Freud, the first scientist to describe the death wish, was completely unable to control his craving for cigars in spite of the fact that he knew the smoke was killing him. Here was certainly the ultimate confirmation of the Freudian doctrine that the irrational forces in man's nature are so strong that the rational forces have little chance against them. An unsuccessfully treated head and neck cancer will usually recur within the first year after treatment and will almost inevitably reappear within the first two years. Obviously a cure had been effected after the first operation in 1923, and a second cure after the 1931 surgery. Had Freud been able to stop smoking during this period, very likely his life would have been prolonged, and he would have been spared the gruesome death from oral cancer. But very few cancer patients are able to give up this powerfully addicting habit.

The Larynx

The larynx, a most important organ composed mainly of cartilage and muscle, has two functions: (1) producing speech by means of the vibrating vocal cords and (2) closing off the oral cavity from the trachea during swallowing to prevent solid material from entering the lungs.

The majority of larynx tumors arise from the surface cells. For unknown reasons, 95 percent of larynx cancer occurs in males, but rarely in black males. The peak incidence is in the fifties and sixties. Like the other head and neck tumors, laryngeal cancer is seen almost exclusively in heavy smokers and chronic alcoholics. A famous case of this tumor—one that changed the history of the twentieth century—serves to illustrate the salient features of the disease.

In the winter of 1887, Crown Prince Friedrich Wilhelm, heir to the throne of Prussia, developed a persistent sore throat. Professor Karl Gerhardt, a Berlin specialist, performed an examination in March and discovered a small growth on the left vocal cord. Six other German doctors also examined the crown prince, and the consensus was firm: the tumor was cancerous and should be removed by an immediate operation. If the patient survived, he would be able to speak only in a hoarse whisper for the rest of his life.

The diagnosis and treatment of diseases of the throat was a relatively new medical specialty in the 1880s. A London singing teacher, Manuel Garcia, had invented the laryngoscope in 1854. Garcia was interested in using the device to observe the vocal cord workings only from a pedagogical standpoint. But when he presented his discovery to the Royal Society in 1855, it attracted the attention of Drs. Ludwig Türck and Johann Czermak of Vienna. Both these men applied the larygoscope independently to diagnostic poblems, and their vituperative debate over the question of "priority" helped to arouse and sustain professional interest in the field.

Once the larynx and its lesions could be observed, procedures were developed to remove laryngeal tumors, which had formerly caused death by suffocation. Surgeons could now cut out small growths with a fairly good chance of success, removing an extra margin of tissue should a malignancy be suspected. To perform this operation on Crown Prince Friedrich Wilhelm, the German government summoned an Englishman, Morrell Mackenzie, Britain's outstanding laryngologist and the foremost throat specialist in Europe.

Mackenzie arrived in Berlin on May 20, 1887. He took a specimen of the growth and sent it to Rudolf Virchow, the leading German pathologist. Unfortunately, Virchow erred in the microscopic diagnosis of the tissue specimen and pronounced it benign. When informed, Mackenzie advised against the operation, suggested that the crown prince come to England for treatment, and predicted a speedy recovery.

The German doctors were distinctily less sanguine, but they could not agree on what should be done. Some advised the operation; others suggested carrying out Mackenzie's treatment in Berlin. Gerhardt wanted Mackenzie himself to treat the patient in the German capital. Whatever was to be done, everyone knew the crown prince's illness had come at a pivotal point in German history.

By the late 1880s, the Prussian imperial family had split into two irreconcilable parts: on the one side, the reactionary old Kaiser Wilhelm I and his grandson, Prince Wilhelm; on the other, the progressive crown prince. Prince Wilhelm had incurred an obstetrical injury at birth, an Erb's palsy, that resulted in a withered left arm. Perhaps to compensate for this deformity, he became arrogant, bombastic, and conceited, and his views grew increasingly reactionary. The sentiments of Friedrich Wilhelm were diametrically opposed; they were liberal, more democratic, and less warlike.

Gerhardt reluctantly agreed that treatment should be given in England. Friedrich Wilhelm was delighted, because he had great taste for ceremony and longed to represent the kaiser at Queen Victoria's jubilee celebration. No one who saw the fifty-five-year-old crown prince riding in the jubilee cavalcade imagined that he was seriously ill. Even the queen, who knew something was wrong, remarked on how healthy and handsome he looked. After the festivities, the crown prince and his wife, Vicky, daughter of Queen Victoria, spent two months in England for Mackenzie's treatment. Everyone was convinced that complete recovery was simply a matter of time. "He is wonderfully better," remarked the queen, and in a rush of premature relief she knighted Mackenzie.

In the autumn Friedrich Wilhelm and his wife left England

and traveled to San Remo on the Mediterranean for the period of convalescence. Meanwhile public opinion in Berlin grew increasingly critical. Some said that the crown prince should return at once; certain liberals feared that Prince Wilhelm was gaining too much influence. Others suspected that Mackenzie was a fraud and that the German doctors' diagnosis of cancer had been correct. Twenty-four hours after the royal couple had settled at San Remo, the worst fears were realized.

Mackenzie, performing a follow-up throat examination, discovered a new growth. The crown prince begged to be told if it was cancer. "I am sorry to say, sir," answered Mackenzie, "it looks very much like it, but it is impossible to be certain." After a moment of silence, the doctor was calmly thanked for his frankness. Only later, alone with his wife, did Friedrich Wilhelm break down and sob bitterly.

There was no doubt that death was imminent. Would the crown prince outlast his ailing father, or would Prince Wilhelm be the next kaiser? The German public whispered a half-forgotten prophecy that Kaiser Wilhelm I would die at ninety-six and be succeeded by a man with one arm. German doctors assured Prince Wilhelm that his father would not live much longer, perhaps allowing Wilhelm II to succeed Wilhelm I.

But the young prince's hopes were in vain. On March 9, 1888, the old kaiser died, two weeks short of turning ninety-one. Friedrich Wilhelm was strolling through the grounds at San Remo when he received the news that he was now Kaiser Friedrich III. Most of his brief reign was spent in bed, and death came on June 15, 1888. Defying his father's instructions, Wilhelm permitted an autopsy to prove publicly that the German doctors' diagnosis of cancer had been right all along.

Doctors today continue to use Manuel Garcia's invention to diagnose laryngeal lesions. The indirect laryngoscope—a light source and a dental mirror—is still the simplest and most expedient tool. In addition, a direct laryngoscopy may be performed by using a long metal tube to look down the throat.

Recently, flexible fiberoptic laryngoscopes have made this process easier. An X-ray examination called a laryngogram requires that iodized oil be introduced into the throat to produce a film of the laryngeal structures.

Could modern medical techniques have saved Friedrich III? The answer is very likely yes. Radiation therapy administered externally is of great value in the treatment of all laryngeal lesions, but especially the early ones such as the Prussian crown prince had. Five-year survival of 85 percent can be expected. Surgical treatment can also be used, but patients will be left permanenly hoarse; radiation rarely produces this complication.

For the more advanced laryngeal cancers, many doctors think that radiation therapy should still be employed as the first means of treatment. A study done by Dr. Steward Lott at Johns Hopkins showed that a large number of such cases could be cured by this modality alone, and the remainder were still good surgical candidates after the X-ray treatments, a notable exception to the rule that curative radiation and surgery are mutually exclusive. When surgery is done, the entire larynx must be removed, leaving the patient voiceless and necessitating respiration through a hole in the neck (a tracheostomy) for the duration of life. Susceptibility to lung infections is also greatly increased after surgical treatment.

Even when radiation is employed on the larynx itself, a surgeon may still want to do a radical neck dissection to remove lymph nodes in the neck. But this is a scarring, often disabling operation. The same result can often be accomplished by radiation therapy to both sides of the neck with far less mutilation.

But the best defense against laryngeal cancer is prevention and early detection. Smokers should kick the habit if they can. Any hoarseness of more than two weeks' duration requires immediate examination of the vocal cords. And before surgery is contemplated, a qualified radiotherapist should be consulted, one preferably at a large university medical center not associated with the ear, nose, and throat specialist who performed the laryngeal examination.

The Paranasal Sinuses

"Product X drains all eight nasal sinuses to relieve a cold's misery!" Everyone is familiar with sinus problems from the familiar television and magazine ads, but what do the sinuses really do? No one is certain. We are only sure that there are four pairs of sinuses, on either side of the skull. The maxillary sinuses, behind the cheeks, are the largest and generally most troublesome. The frontal sinuses, just above the eyes, are also prone to infections. The ethmoid and sphenoid sinuses are located more deeply within the skull and are heard from less often.

Paranasal sinus tumors make up 3 percent of all head and neck cancers. Women are affected slightly more often in this region than in other parts of the head and neck. For reasons that remain obscure, the incidence is much higher in Orientals, comprising 50 percent of all their head and neck lesions in one study. Of all the sinuses, the maxillary sinus predominates as a cancer site, harboring 90 percent of all tumors. The sphenoid sinuses rank a distant second with over 9 percent. Cancer rarely appears in the frontal or ethmoid sinuses. A famous case of maxillary sinus cancer in President Grover Cleveland illustrates some typical features.

President Cleveland developed the first symptom, a rough spot in the roof of his mouth, during the financial panic of 1893. Because of the perilous state of the country, surgery to remove the tumor was secretly performed on a yacht in the middle of New York Harbor. Two operations were necessary, but the president made a complete recovery and lived for another fifteen years.

President Cleveland's presenting sign for sinus cancer, a growth into the oral cavity, is seen in 20 percent of all such patients. Other signs are bulging of an eye, paralysis of an eye muscle, toothache, loosening of a tooth, or denture discomfort.

Sinus tumors today are usually treated by an external approach; in contrast, Cleveland's tumor was removed from inside his mouth. If the lesion is found to be growing into the eye socket, the eye must be removed. Before or following surgery, external radiation therapy is administered. Five-year survival is currently 20 to 30 percent, but if the tumor is invading bone, the chances for cure are poorer.

Nasal Fossa and Nasopharynx

Cancer of the nasal fossa, the interior of the nose, is quite rare. The first symptom is usually bloody nasal discharge and breathing obstruction. Diagnosis is made by using an instrument, the nasal speculum, to inspect the interior of the nose and facilitate removal of tissue for microscopic examination. The best mode of treatment is radiation therapy because cure rates are comparable to surgery with a much better cosmetic result. Surgical intervention is warranted only for those tumors that are resistant to X rays. Five-year survival of 80 percent is expected.

The nasopharynx is an open chamber the size of a matchbox that is situated behind the nasal fossa below the base of the skull and above the soft palate. Tumors here are also uncommon, comprising less than 1 percent of all cancer in the United States. For reasons that are unclear, Chinese people are especially susceptible. The onset of the disease is generally at about the age of fifty, with men being afflicted twice as often as women.

Typically, the first symptom is the development of a peculiar nasal twang to the voice or a nasal obstruction. Over a third of the patients will have involvement of the cranial nerves by tumor, leading to paralysis of swallowing, facial, or eye muscles. A third of the cases will complain of pain because of tumor destruction of bone at the base of the skull. Enlarged lymph nodes perceived as hard lumps in the neck are also common.

Diagnosis is made with a device called the nasopharyngoscope, a small periscope that is inserted through the nose and is capable of visualizing the nasopharynx. An indirect look at some of the same structures can be obtained with a good light source and an angled dental mirror held at the back of the throat. X-ray films of the skull are particularly valuable for revealing the extent of bone destruction.

Radiation therapy is the only accepted form of treatment for nasopharyngeal tumors. Surgery should never be used because of the technical difficulties attending the complete removal of the tumor. Superior results can be obtained using radiotherapy exclusively. Unfortunately, overall five-year survival for adequately treated cases is about 25 percent, principally because these tumors tend to spread very early. One special type of lesion, the lymphoma, has a more favorable outlook.

The Lips

Lip cancers account for a sizable proportion of all head and neck malignancies—more than 15 percent. Ninety percent of the lesions occur in males, almost always on the lower lip. Black men are rarely affected. The incidence increases after the age of forty. Exposure to sun and wind or the chronic irritation produced by a pipe stem are common causative factors.

Most characteristically a lip cancer is first observed to be a painless sore that is present for more than two weeks. Leukoplakia, a premalignant condition, is observed as a persistent whitish patch. Diagnosis is direct: a small piece of tissue removed for microscopic examination is all that is required.

Removal of leukoplakia consists of a superficial scraping called a "lip shave." Small lip cancers can be treated with either surgery or radiation therapy, but for more extensive lesions radiation is the treatment of choice because the cosmetic results are far superior to those of the most expert surgery. Five-year survival approaches 90 percent in uncomplicated cases.

The Salivary Glands

The salivary glands produce saliva necessary for digestion and for maintenance of the oral cavity. The importance of saliva can be demonstrated after radiation has been administered to the head. If too large a dose has been received by the salivary glands, salivary secretion is altered, and the mouth becomes dry. A rapid decaying of the teeth (radiation caries) occurs because the normal saliva is vital in preserving dental health.

Three-fourths of salivary gland tumors are benign in adults. Children are more likely to have malignant lesions. Of the three pairs of glands, the parotid is most commonly affected. Just in front of and below the ear, the parotid occupies a very sensitive position. Passing through the glandular substance is the facial nerve, which controls all of the facial muscles, including those necessary to blink the eye.

Most salivary tumors are first noted as a mass or lump just below and in front of the ear. If the tumor is benign, growth will be at a slow and steady pace, there will be no pain, and the lump will be rubbery in consistency and movable under the skin. Malignant tumors grow rapidly, are frequently painful, stony hard, and fixed; in addition, the facial nerve is often affected by parotid tumors, producing a facial palsy. With the ability to blink impaired, the cornea of the eye becomes ulcerated, and vision is lost.

Diagnosis of these tumors is usually made by observation alone. Biopsy removal of tissue for microscopic examination is not advisable because of the propensity of the tumor cells to be spread. A chest X ray is made to inspect the lungs, a common site of metastasis for the malignant lesions.

Surgery is the first recourse in all small tumors and in tumors not obviously malignant. Because many benign lesions are encapsulated, apparently completely separated from the gland substance, an inexperienced or unknowledgeable surgeon may attempt to shell the tumor out like a pea from a pod; this often leads to recurrent growth of the few cells left behind. The proper surgical therapy is complete removal of the lobe of the gland containing the tumor; if this is carefully performed, the facial nerve can be spared. Radiation therapy is used for recurrent or inoperable cancers and for cancers incompletely removed at surgery.

In addition to the three distinct pairs of salivary glands, there is salivary tissue located in the palate, tongue, nasal cavity, and other sites. This tissue can give rise to the same types of tumors found in the salivary glands themselves, but such lesions are seen much less frequently than parotid gland tumors. A higher proportion of these rarer tumors is malignant.

After a benign tumor has been properly removed, a recurrence should appear in only 2 percent of cases. The improper method mentioned—shelling out the tumor—can lead to a 20 percent recurrence rate. One quarter of recurrences will be malignant, and one-third will be incurable. Five-year survival after treatment for a primary malignant tumor varies from 15 percent for highly malignant lesions to 85 percent for low-grade malignancies.

12 Tumors of
Bone and Soft Tissue

Bone

Compared to tumors in other sites, tumors originating in bone are rather rare. The highest incidence is during adolescence, three per hundred thousand, which is roughly comparable to the overall incidence of Hodgkin's disease. This figure falls to two per million at age thirty-five, then slowly rises until at age sixty it is comparable to that at adolescence.

What causes bone cancer? One suspect factor must be rapid growth. Children from birth to age eighteen with osteogenic sarcoma, the most common childhood bone tumor, have been found to be significantly taller than a hospital control group with nonbone tumors. Bone tumors of children appear commonly in those parts of the bone that are developing most quickly. Patients with Paget's disease, a disorder of older adults in which the bones grow abnormally and become deformed, have a 10 percent chance of being afflicted with osteogenic sarcoma.

Another cancer-causing factor is radiation. One group of young women employed to paint radium watch dials moistened their brushes in their mouths. Many later died of osteogenic sarcoma. And infants receiving external radiation for treatment of retinoblastoma, an eye tumor, may later develop osteogenic sarcoma of the skull.

A typical case of childhood bone tumor occurred in the son of the United States Senator from Massachusetts.

Edward M. Kennedy Jr., 12, was highly competitive and

athletic. He played on the football team at the Washington area's exclusive St. Alban's School.... He rafted down the Colorado River with his father ... played a vigorous game of tennis on the family courts at McLean, Virginia, and skied at Sun Valley....

Young Teddy's ordeal began [December 1973] ... when he told his father that his leg hurt and that there was a swelling below the knee. The Senator, who is chairman of the Subcommittee on Health, called a committee consultant, who in turn recommended a specialist: Dr. George Hyatt, a professor of surgery at Georgetown University Hospital. Admitted to the hospital for a biopsy and other tests on a Friday morning, Teddy was examined, released for the weekend, and sent back to school the following Monday. But Tuesday the results of the tests had come back from the lab; the youngster had chondrosarcoma, a fast growing cancer of the cartilage [that is about half as common as osteogenic sarcoma]....

Teddy's mother Joan was summoned home from Europe; the diagnosis and the fact that amputation was necessary were kept from the youngster until she arrived. Reporters... were asked to delay publication of the news. "We didn't want him to hear on the radio or see in the paper that he had cancer," said a family friend....

Friends say that the child took it well. "You could tell by the Senator's reaction when it was over—he was a mirror of how the boy reacted," said one Kennedy intimate. "He was grim but you could tell things had gone about as well as something like that can go."

The hour-long operation, the following Saturday morning, appeared to go equally well. Doctors cut back the skin, muscle, and other tissue ... to form a well-padded stump.... A day after the operation, he left his bed briefly and read some of the thousands of letters and telegrams wishing him a speedy recovery.[1]

---

1. Reprinted by permission from *Time,* The Weekly Newsmagazine; Copyright Time, Inc. 1973.

As in Teddy Kennedy's case, surgery is considered the definitive treatment for both osteogenic sarcoma and chondrosarcoma, which is much slower growing and has a better outlook. Ewing's sarcoma, a highly malignant and rapidly growing tumor of childhood, is never treated surgically because of its almost total incurability; the tumor's high sensitivity to radiation makes this mode of therapy valuable for symptomatic relief.

A special form of anticancer drug therapy, rescue therapy, is coming into wider use, especially in children. The drug methotrexate is given in enormous and ordinarily fatal doses, but before death can occur massive amounts of the vitamin-antidote citrovorum factor are administered. Teddy Kennedy received this treatment.

Besides the malignant tumors of bone, benign tumors are also encountered. An example is the giant cell tumor. Occurring commonly at about the age of thirty, this tumor is frequently found around the knee. The symptoms are very similar to those that Teddy Kennedy's chondrosarcoma produced, but since growth is slower they might be ignored for a longer period of time. Treatment is surgical; an attempt is made to scrape out the entire tumor and pack the resulting cavity with bone chips. Unfortunately, this procedure must sometimes be performed more than once, for these lesions tend to recur. Radiation therapy may be administered after the first recurrence, but with a certain element of risk—the X rays sometimes cause the tumor to become malignant.

Statistical survival percentages are more unreliable in bone tumors than in other types of cancer. The evaluation and classification of these lesions is highly variable and specialized, making the results of many series of cases doubtful. The site of the tumor greatly affects survival. For example, a tumor of the pelvis is worse than one of the same type occurring in the hand. Each patient must be treated individually after a full study of his specific lesion. Malignant bone tumors are far from hopeless, and all deserve aggressive therapy.

Soft Tissue

Soft-tissue cancer, like bone cancer, is an uncommon form of malignancy, comprising only 0.3–0.4 percent of all cancers. Classified as sarcomas because of their connective tissue origin, the majority arise from smooth muscle, voluntary muscle, fat, cartilage, or blood vessels. Any site within the body where this normal tissue is present may be a point of origin. The rate of growth of these cancers is entirely unpredictable.

Age at onset is characteristic of the particular tumor. For example, fibrosarcomas, originating from fibrous tissue, occur at all ages without sex predilection. Liposarcomas, arising from fat cells, are found predominantly between the ages of forty and sixty. Rhabdomyosarcomas, which develop from muscle, are found at any age but most commonly in the twenties and thirties; a peculiar form of rhabdomyosarcoma occurs in the eye muscles of young children.

The cause of soft-tissue sarcomas is unknown. Though these tumors occasionally grow from old scars, trauma has never been definitely incriminated. Intensive irradiation is more suspect; when given for nonmalignant conditions, such as tuberculosis of the skin or thyroid disease, it has produced fibrosarcomas. A third possibility is obstruction. After radical mastectomy, an arm will frequently swell because of lymphatic blockage; a rare soft-tissue tumor, lymphangiosarcoma, has been reported in a few of these patients. A fourth cause may be Von Recklinghausen's disease. This malady is associated with many benign tumors of nerve sheaths, and these sometimes become malignant.

The first sign of a soft-tissue sarcoma is usually a mass that grows and often develops a hard consistency. Symptoms may be produced by pressure on nerves or blood vessels. Some soft-tissue cancers may interfere with visceral structures. The result—obstruction of the bowel or urinary tract. Because these tumors often grow deep within the body, early detection is difficult.

Surgery is the definitive treatment for those soft-tissue sarcomas that may be completely removed. But such cancers are among the most difficult to control locally because they spread impalpably far from their point of origin. Recurrence rates, even in the best series, are about 30 percent, and the appearance of a local recurrence doubles the probability that the patient will die from the tumor. For this reason, an extensive surgical procedure is the most prudent method of therapy; but unfortunately, since many sarcomas begin in a limb, this means amputation.

Radiation therapy alone is not always effective as a curative treatment for sarcomas, particularly large, bulky ones. Reports have appeared of dramatic resolution and regression of some lesions after X-ray therapy, but no one can say in advance which tumors will respond and which won't. Under these circumstances, most physicians consider radiation only a useful adjunct to surgery. At the Maimonides Medical Center in Brooklyn, however, sarcoma patients received radiation combined with the drug methotrexate. Survival time was extended from two to nineteen months, and of seven patients treated, three were alive and without evidence of disease after forty-eight, forty-five, and twenty-nine months. A rapidly changing field, drug therapy combined with radiation may be expected to play an expanding role in this form of cancer.

13 Tumors of Children

Retinoblastoma

This hereditary malignant eye tumor occurs once in every twenty thousand births in the United States; about two hundred new cases are seen yearly. For reasons that are unclear, incidence has doubled within the past twenty years. This once rare lesion is now the second most common malignancy of childhood.

The only known causative factor in retinoblastoma is heredity. True, 94 percent of cases appear sporadically, without a family history, but at least 25 percent of these are genetic mutations transmittable to offspring. Six percent of all cases run in families and have a dominant genetic pattern: if one parent was affected, the child will have a 50 percent chance of getting the tumor; if both parents were affected, the chances are 75 percent. Healthy parents with a single affected child have a 6 percent chance of producing another child with the same tumor.

In sporadic cases, the first symptoms of retinoblastoma are usually noticed by the mother. An affected infant will characteristically lose the normal deep black pupil, which is replaced by a whitish-appearing "cat's eye." The interference with vision due to growth of the tumor within the eye may cause the eyes to cross, or abnormally high fluid pressure and glaucoma can appear when normal outflow paths are blocked. When retinoblastoma has already been detected in one eye, there should be follow-up examinations of the opposite eye and of the eyes of siblings so as to reveal any subsequent tumors at a much earlier stage.

The first cures of retinoblastoma were achieved by Dr. A. B. Reese with radiation therapy in 1933. Today radiation and surgery are used in combination. If only one eye is involved, surgical removal of the eye is considered the best form of treatment. If both eyes are involved, the worse eye is removed, the better eye irradiated. Small tumors in both eyes should receive only radiation therapy. Concomitant administration of the drug TEM (triethylenemelamine) is believed to improve chances for survival.

Why is radiation not the sole treatment in all cases? Retinoblastomas can be eradicated with small or moderate doses, but unwanted complications may be produced. While the normal retina easily withstands the necessary X-ray treatments, the lens of the eye does not. In spite of attempts to shield or protect this structure, radiation cataract is often the price paid for cure of the tumor. Fortunately, such cataracts can be removed easily. A more serious complication of X-ray treatment is the growth-retarding effect on the bones around the eye. Considerable facial asymmetry may result when a child under two years of age is treated. In the past, radiation has also been responsible for the late appearance of malignant bone and muscle tumors; the lower doses given today have resulted in far fewer of these lesions.

The chances of survival and good vision depend heavily on how early the tumor is first diagnosed. When untreated, retinoblastoma is almost invariably fatal. With therapy, however, the overall mortality rate drops to 20 percent, though each individual's chances are heavily dependent upon the size and location of the tumor when treatment is started. The lesion can be extensive in one eye before the patient exhibits any signs or is brought for examination, a fact that is mainly responsible for the 20 percent mortality rate. Nearly all fatalities are observed within two years of onset.

Occasionally, one painful decision must be made by physician and parents: Should the child's life be risked by retaining the second eye harboring tumor and treating it with radiation? Or is the second eye best removed, thereby protecting life at the expense of vision? This choice is one of the most difficult in all of medicine.

Wilms' Tumor

Wilms' tumor, a malignant lesion of the kidney, is the most common cancerous tumor of childhood. The origin is believed to be groups of primitive cells in the kidney. Sixty-five percent of all cases occur before the age of three, 75 percent before the age of five. Boys and girls are equally affected, with both kidneys harboring tumor in 7.2 percent of all cases.

A Wilms' tumor is most commonly first detected as an abdominal mass palpated by a mother bathing a child. In an infant, an abdominal mass most likely represents blockage of a kidney, but in somewhat older children malignancy becomes more probable. Other signs of Wilms' tumor are blood in the urine, pain, and symptoms of elevated blood pressure, especially headache.

Intravenous pyelography, an X-ray test to visualize the kidneys, is the most valuable diagnostic tool when Wilms' tumor is suspected. Recently, a technique using high-frequency sound waves (ultrasound) has been employed in detecting kidney lesions. The new CAT scanners will undoubtedly prove even more effective. A chest X ray is also important, for the tumor frequently spreads to the lungs.

Once the presence of Wilms' tumor has been documented, the affected kidney should be removed immediately. Postoperative radiation therapy is of great value because of this cancer's exquisite sensitivity to X rays. Actinomycin D, a toxic antibiotic first used in these cases by Dr. Sidney Farber at the Boston Children's Hospital, has produced a dramatic increase in survivals. Even children with formerly incurable tumor metastases in both lungs are now being saved in 58 percent of cases with the combination of actinomycin D and pulmonary irradiation.

Two-year survival of 40 percent without the drug more than doubles to 89 percent when it is used.

Neuroblastoma

At least 8 to 10 percent of the malignant tumors of childhood are neuroblastomas. In one study, Dr. Sidney Farber found 40 cases among 300 childhood cancers. One-third of all these lesions arise in infants less than a year old; the incidence drops to 15 percent per year thereafter until the age of six or seven. Heredity also plays a role. In the *New England Journal of Medicine,* Dr. J. Chatlen reported on a series of cases occurring in siblings.

The neuroblastoma develops from primitive nervous tissue, the neural crest tissue, that forms the sympathetic nervous system. These are the nerves necessary for "fight or flight." Tumors may arise in any sympathetic nerve from the neck to the pelvis but most commonly grow from tissue around the kidney, especially the adrenal gland.

Most neuroblastomas are highly malignant, tending to spread early and widely to bone, liver, skin, bone marrow, and lung. One strange aspect of this cancer is its behavior in children under three months of age; a certain number of these lesions become benign and cause no further difficulty.

A child with a neuroblastoma will typically be noted by the mother to have a fixed, lobulated, painless mass in the neck or abdomen. Because some tumors manufacture the compounds epinephrine and norepinephrine, which cause the blood pressure to rise, the first complaint may be a symptom of high blood pressure, such as headache. Less common signs are bulging of an eye, pallor, fever, weakness, weight loss, cough, or shortness of breath.

Diagnosis of neuroblastoma is made, for the most part, with X rays or chemical tests. Often the lesions will be detected on X ray because they displace a kidney or cause changes in a bone. In up to 80 percent of cases, the epinephrine and norepinephrine synthesized by the tumor are converted to the compound VMA (vanillomandelic acid), which can be identified in the child's urine with a simple laboratory test, the La Brosse Spot Test. Also available for mass screening are paper dip strips like those used by diabetics for testing urinary glucose.

The best hope for cure of neuroblastoma is offered by total surgical excision. If there is no evidence that tumor has spread to bone, even a partial excision is worthwhile. But if metastasis can be documented, no surgery should be attempted. Neuroblastomas are very sensitive to radiation, cures having been achieved by this method alone even after metastatic spread to the liver. Some cancer specialists think that X rays should be delivered to the tumor bed after a partial excision, but this is disputed. Two drugs, cyclophosphamide and vincristine, are capable of producing tumor regression in half of all cases, but this response is of short duration. Newer compounds may prove to be of more value.

Many researchers studying neuroblastoma have concluded that a therapy activating or increasing the body's immune response may ultimately prove most effective. Spontaneous regression has been documented in this tumor more frequently than in any other form of cancer, with as many as 1 to 2 percent of cases disappearing by themselves. Even after an incomplete surgical excision, some tumors vanish, most commonly in children under two years of age. No doubt immunity plays a large part in these regressions, but the exact mechanism remains obscure. Perhaps in the future an effective form of immunotherapy may be devised.

Age seems to be the greatest factor influencing survival. Infants with neuroblastoma present at birth can be cured in almost all cases with proper treatment. Children under one year of age have a 60 percent chance of cure, whereas those older than two have a 15 percent survival rate. Freedom from tumor fourteen months after therapy is considered a cure by most authorities.

Other Children's Tumors

Rhabdomyosarcoma, a muscle tumor, affects children as well as adults. This highly malignant lesion may arise from almost any voluntary muscle, usually in a child between the ages of two and six. While attempts at surgical cure have not met with stunning success, combinations of surgery, radiotherapy, and drug therapy offer more promise; these are now being studied in a number of hospitals.

Hepatoma is a highly malignant liver tumor, fortunately rare in childhood. It is seldom seen in children older than three. Cures may be produced by surgical excision in 30 to 50 percent of cases. The combined use of surgery, radiotherapy, and drug therapy is now being investigated.

Teratoma is an unusual form of cancer, which can contain any type of body tissue—nerve, muscle, cartilage, or primitive cells. Occurring once in forty thousand live births, these lesions are most commonly found at the base of the spine, though they may be in the space between the lungs (the mediastinum), in the ovaries, in the testes, near the kidneys, or in the mouth. The benign teratomas are more commonly seen in females, while the malignant ones have an equal sex distribution. Surgical removal is the only effective form of treatment. More than 80 percent of patients will survive the benign lesions, but fewer than 15 percent the malignant ones.

14 Tumors of the Thyroid and Adrenal Glands

Thyroid

The butterfly-shaped thyroid gland sits astride the neck just below the Adam's apple. Intimately concerned with the regulation of metabolism, the thyroid cells produce two iodine-containing hormones: thyroxine and triiodothyronine. A healthy thyroid acts like an officer in the military chain of command, receiving chemical orders from the chief of staff, the pituitary, and performing accordingly. Sometimes, however, the thyroid ignores the pituitary's physiologic messenger, the thyroid-stimulating hormone (TSH); a metabolically chaotic situation, hyperthyroidism, is the result. But cancer is rarely a problem here; fewer than one in five thousand overactive glands will be found malignant.

The cause of thyroid cancer is unknown. In animals, severe iodine restriction is capable of producing cancer. An analogous situation in humans is the formation of goiter, a nodular enlargement of the gland seen commonly in persons who ingest too little iodine or too much cabbage and grape seed. A large goiter in a woman's neck was once considered an attribute of beauty; doctors now know that 6 to 10 percent of goiters are cancerous.

Radiation, like iodine restriction, is another factor capable of inducing thyroid cancer, especially when administered to a young individual. A significant number of malignancies have appeared in children and young adults who received therapeutic radiation to shrink a large thymus or large tonsils. And many Japanese exposed to the intensive radiation of the Hiroshima bombing have gone on to develop thyroid cancer. Two less well-defined factors influencing thyroid cancer are sex and heredity. Women are vastly more susceptible than men to all forms of thyroid disease, and three to four times as vulnerable to cancers. Though most thyroid cancer is believed not to be inherited, one form called medullary carcinoma may be in some cases.

Of the twenty-five new thyroid cancers per million people that begin each year, most are first noted as a solitary thyroid nodule. Such a lump may be initially seen or felt by the patient, or it may be detected by a physician on a routine examination. Fortunately, very few nodules are malignant. One study found that 15 to 20 percent of solitary nodules are cancerous, but other thyroid specialists put this same figure at less than 1 percent.

Two types of nodules may be identified in the thyroid: functioning and nonfunctioning. A functioning nodule is usually an encapsulated aggregation of thyroid tissue called an adenoma, rarely malignant, and capable of producing thyroid hormones without the stimulation of the pituitary's chemical messenger, TSH. Often the excess hormones will stop the pituitary from sending out TSH, thus "turning off" the entire thyroid gland except for the nodule. Patients with such a lesion may or may not have enough thyroid hormone to generate the symptoms and signs of hyperthyroidism: bulging eyes, rapid pulse, sweaty skin, and heat intolerance. Treatment for this condition is administration of radioactive iodine, which is accumulated preferentially by the overactive adenoma and subsequently destroys it.

A nonfunctioning nodule may be composed of various elements: (1) abnormal but nonmalignant thyroid tissue; (2) cystic fluid, hemorrhaged blood, or calcium; or (3) rarely, malignant thyroid tissue or metastatic cancerous tissue from a lung, breast, or kidney tumor. Especially suspect of malignancy is a solitary thyroid nodule in a male under age thirty.

How does a doctor determine whether a nodule is functioning or nonfunctioning? A very small dose of radioactive iodine is administered as a pill by mouth. The iodine is then taken up preferentially by thyroid tissue, and a device called a rectilinear scanner is used to form a paper or film image of the thyroid gland from the radioactivity emitted. Those nodules that take up iodine and emit radiation are said to be functioning. Recently, a technique called ultrasound imaging, which makes use of high-frequency sound waves, has shown promise in differentiating cysts from solid tumors.

Four types of cancer originate in the thyroid and may be identified microscopically by cellular architecture. Papillary carcinoma, the most common form, is responsible for more than 50 percent of all adult and 70 percent of all childhood cases. Tending to remain localized for many years, this tumor does not cause death by spread to lymph nodes and lungs before age forty in most cases. Follicular carcinoma, which makes up 30 percent of all thyroid cancers, usually appears between the ages of thirty through fifty and may be more malignant than papillary cancer. Medullary carcinoma is a solid, rather slowly growing lesion, sometimes associated with an adrenal tumor called pheochromocytoma. Anaplastic carcinoma is one of the most malignant tumors known; most patients with this disease die within one to two years.

Early treatment should be the rule in all cases of thyroid cancer, though the value of surgery is sometimes questioned. Total removal of the thyroid is practiced for papillary, follicular, and medullary cancers, with excision of neck lymph nodes as well. But several good studies of papillary cancer conclude that the course of the disease is not altered by the extent of the operation; life is instead prolonged by orally administering thyroid hormones after surgery to stop the pituitary from making TSH and stimulating further tumor growth.

Patients under age forty with papillary cancer have the best chance for long-term survival. Even distant metastases in such organs as bone and liver respond well to radioactive iodine therapy. The proof: investigators have noticed that institutions reporting a relatively large number of thyroid cancers also report a relatively small number of deaths and few autopsies of thyroid cancer pations. Obviously many such patients live for long periods with their disease, finally going on to die of an unrelated condition.

While no disputes occur over the surgical removal of a malignant thyroid or a suspicious solitary nodule, some debate can arise over how to treat a benign goiter. Surgeons are often anxious to operate on these lesions, but this treatment has drawbacks:

1. Thyroid hormone must be taken orally for the duration of life if the entire thyroid gland is removed.
2. A vital structure in the neck, the recurrent laryngeal nerve, is occasionally severed during surgery, leaving the patient permanently hoarse.
3. The parathyroid glands, four small structures in the periphery of the thyroid tissue, are essential for the regulation of calcium metabolism. When these are accidentally removed with the thyroid, a life-threatening, chemical imbalance occurs, which is difficult to treat.

Adrenal

Thomas Addison, a brilliant diagnostician and pathology lecturer of London's Guy's Hospital, first recognized in 1855 that the adrenal glands were necessary for life. During his own lifetime, Addison's findings were regarded as a mere scientific curiosity, and he himself was seen as a haughty, repellent, unsuccessful practitioner. Attaching little importance to "drugging," the famous physician sometimes forgot to prescribe medication at all. Perhaps this was fortunate; his most famous concoction, "Addison's pill," containing calomel, digitalis, and

squills, was discarded years ago as worthless. But adrenal insufficiency, or Addison's disease, is recognized today as a specific malady. A famous case was President John F. Kennedy.
The adrenal gland consists of two portions: an outer cortex and an inner medulla. Two steroid hormones, cortisol and aldosterone, are produced by the cortex. Cortisol provides resistance to a wide variety of stresses and maintains the activity of a number of enzyme systems. Aldosterone enables the withstanding of salt restriction. When an animal is deprived of the adrenal cortex, circulatory collapse and death result. The adrenal medulla, not as vital to life as the cortex, is part of the sympathetic nervous system, the mediator of the "fight or flight" response. Epinephrine (adrenalin) and norepinephrine, the medullary hormones, ready the body for bursts of strenuous activity.

Cancer of the adrenal cortex is a rare, highly malignant tumor usually diagnosed only when advanced and incurable. The lesion may be a large, nonfunctioning mass that encroaches on neighboring structures, or it may consist of functioning, hormone-producing cells. Various abnormalities will develop due to the hormone excesses:

1. Superfluous cortisol leads to Cushing's syndrome. Patients show poor wound healing, a moon face, a buffalo-humped back, stretch marks on the skin, and bone demineralization.

2. When androgen, the male hormone, is synthesized by a tumor in a woman, masculinization results, with deepening of voice, clitoral enlargement, growth of beard, male pattern baldness, and increased sex drive.

3. If estrogen, the female hormone, is produced by a tumor in a man, it generates breast enlargement, loss of sex drive, and shriveled testes.

4. Excessive aldosterone from some lesions causes high blood pressure.

Not all adrenal cortical tumors are malignant. Benign growths are capable of producing the above manifestations, but a return to normal takes place after the lesion is removed. The same may be said for tumors of the medulla, and a much larger proportion is benign.

The two most common medullary tumors are the ganglioneuroma and the pheochromocytoma. The ganglioneuroma is slow growing and usually produces no symptoms except those relating to its size. The pheochromocytoma is capable of pouring out intermittent bursts of epinephrine and norepinephrine. Patients experience paroxysms of sweating, weakness, facial pallor, elevated blood pressure, and rapid heartbeat. Such attacks may occur many times daily over a period of years and be erroneously attributed to a neurotic personality. Both pheochromocytomas and ganglioneuromas are occasionally found outside the adrenal medulla in other parts of the body.

Two diagnostic tools are used most commonly to diagnose adrenal lesions: X rays and chemical analyses. Since the adrenals are directly above the kidneys, a tumor will often displace a kidney downward. Intravenous pyelography, an X-ray examination capable of displaying the kidneys, can demonstrate the displacement. Angiography, a technique that displays blood vessels, may indicate abnormal arteries or veins supplying one adrenal. Retroperitoneal pneumography, a painful and much talked about but seldom used examination, requires the introtroduction of air to allow the adrenals to be outlined on an X-ray film.

The chemical analyses are most often performed on urine collections made over a twenty-four–hour period. Abnormally high levels of steroid compounds are indicative of an abnormality, though conditions other than adrenal cortical tumor can cause this finding. Excess VMA (vanillomandelic acid), a metabolic byproduct of epinephrine, suggests the presence of pheochromocytoma.

The best treatment for a benign adrenal tumor is surgical removal. Radiotherapy may be given to malignancies, but its value is uncertain. Some drugs, especially a new agent, mitotane, might be worthwhile treatment, but not enough data exist to be sure. Good studies of survival after treated adrenal cancer are simply not available, so any predictions are impossible. Cancer specialists also are unable to say whether a hormone-producing tumor has a better outlook than a non-hormone-producing one.

15 Cancer and Baloney: Management Methods of Dubious Value

Cancer is the most frightening medical diagnosis that can be made; the patient is alarmed, the family is jolted, and sometimes the physician, as well, is scared. Several studies have shown that many doctors and medical students have little faith in our ability to cure cancer, in spite of the two million cancer patients healed annually by conventional medical methods. This terror and suffering associated with cancer—especially incurable cases—allows the propagation of worthless cancer remedies.

Worthless remedies often receive their biggest boost from controversy, because controversy is news. Confrontations between the medical "establishment" and those who oppose it make good reading, good viewing, and stimulating conversation. Though the newspapers, television networks, and book and magazine publishers spend much time telling people about quackery, this negative information sometimes has a promotional effect by putting the quack and his cure in the public eye.

Can worthless remedies ever be done away with? Not likely. Certainly legislation is not the answer; the threat of being branded a criminal might deter a quack, but not the man who believes in his method.

Better communication between doctors and patients is needed. Almost every cancer patient who chooses an unconventional method of treatment has at some point consulted his own physician, according to Dr. Arthur Holleb of the American Cancer Society. A doctor's honest, informed answers to a patient's questions about an unproven or worthless method of treatment can often help the patient see how the facts have been twisted or fragmented. But indifference, ignorance, or hesitancy reinforce the patient's interest in what he heard or read about the unconventional treatment. A number of unproven or worthless cancer management methods are presented here. No patient should lose precious time with any of them.

The Krebiozen Controversy

Some time toward the end of the Second World War, a Yugoslavian refugee physician, Dr. Stevan Durovic, with his lawyer brother, Marko, established the Instituto Biologica Duga in Buenos Aires. Little is known of the brothers' activities in Argentina. Arriving in the United States in 1949, Dr. Durovic brought with him a substance he called Kositerin, alleged to have been isolated from beef blood and used in the treatment of high blood pressure. Dr. Roscoe Miller of Northwestern University, who was first consulted, failed to find the compound effective but referred Durovic to Dr. Andrew Conway Ivy.

The fifty-six-year-old Ivy, vice-president of the University of Illinois, was one of the foremost physiologists in the United States. His studies of the gastrointestinal tract, the gallbladder, the liver, and peptic ulcer disease were considered scientific classics, procuring his appointment as distinguished clinical professor and head of the department of physiology at Illinois. Ivy's prestige in the scientifc community was fated to give Krebiozen its greatest boost.

At his first meeting with Stevan Durovic, Ivy showed no interest in Kositerin. But the ever resourceful Durovic just happened to have with him two grams of a second wonder drug, substance X, extracted from the blood of two thousand Argentinian horses inoculated with *Actinomyces bovis,* a disease-producting fungus. What powers did this magical medicine have? Within six months of treatment, said Durovic, twelve dogs and cats had been cured of cancer; five others were improved.

Ivy was intrigued. Substance X certainly fit with views the eminent physiologist himself held on chemical growth-controlling substances present in the body. In fact, the basic concept that there must be internal control of growth was not unique with Ivy. This notion has been shared by many cancer researchers and has formed the basis of much commendable investigation. The strangest aspect of the Krebiozen story is the alacrity with which Dr. Andrew Conway Ivy—a man who had spent a distinguished scientific career testing the validity of experimental data—accepted Durovic's studies of this worthless medicine.

Specifically, Ivy had not been told the name of the fungus or how the extract was made—all "commercial secrets," Durovic claimed. The shabby experimental protocols, the unsupervised nature of the work, the limited number of animals and questionable observations: any of these should have aroused the suspicions of even a sixth-grade science student.

"I will be the first next to Dr. Durovic, the first human being who has taken the medicine," said the renowned physiologist. And without previously having heard of Durovic as a scientist, without having seen analyses or manufacturing records, without knowing what was in the ampules of oily liquid, Dr. Andrew Conway Ivy, professor of physiology at the University of Illinois, injected himself with Krebiozen.

Nothing happened. The professor survived and was elated. To further verify safety, Ivy tested the compound in a close associate, Louis R. Krasno, M.D., Ph.D., and a large dog. Both showed no ill effects. With still no thought that Krebiozen might be a hoax, Ivy injected the first cancer patient on August 20, 1949. Clinical trials were continued by colleagues and hopeful physicians in the following months.

On March 27, 1951, Ivy decided to announce his findings, but, in violation of the usual principles of medical ethics, he did not do so to a scientific audience. A press conference was held in Chicago's elegant Drake Hotel, to which the science writers of the four local papers, the mayor, two U.S. senators, and potential financial supporters were invited, in addition to several physicians. The results released were dramatic: of twenty-two patients treated with Krebiozen, only eight were dead according to the table in a booklet distributed at the meeting, but in not a single instance was cancer listed as the cause of death. The actual outcome of the tests, unfortunately, was quite different from what Ivy and Durovic proclaimed.

At his trial fourteen years later, Ivy testified that in reality all eight deceased patients had died with and of cancer. Two more of the twenty-two patients had also died, one seven days and one two days prior to the meeting, both from cancer. One was described in the summary as having made "dramatic clinical improvement. Now working all day without opiates. Patient had to be carried, couldn't walk." The physician of this patient, Dr. William F. Phillips, attended the meeting at the Drake Hotel. So did Dr. John F. Pick, whose own wife, the ninth dead patient, had expired seven days previously from breast cancer. Nonetheless, Mrs. Pick's description in the summary was allowed to stand: "had much pain and mild [jaundice]. Local and abdominal metastases have regressed; much improvement." Ivy, who certainly knew of Mrs. Pick's death, did not mention it at the meeting. And because no one asked whether the patients listed were living or dead, Ivy later testified, he did not believe he was obliged to volunteer the information.

Despite considerable skepticism, great scientific excitement was generated by the initial report on Krebiozen. Cancer research centers and universities attempted to confirm Ivy's findings, but to no avail. Nine institutions found the medicine ineffective. Trials at a tenth hospital initially suggested some activity, but upon reappraising their work, the investigators felt there was no evidence Krebiozen was of value in the treatment of cancer and so discontinued the study.

On October 27, 1951, a "Status Report on Krebiozen" was published in the *Journal of the American Medical Association*. The paper consisted of an analysis of the protocols of 100 cases that had been treated by seven investigators selected because of their experience in the diagnosis and therapy of cancer.

Ninety-eight patients showed no improvement after the treatment. Before the article appeared, Ivy had been counseled by a scientist friend that his position was mistaken, that the data reported at the Drake Hotel press conference were not supportable, that no expert confirmation of the findings would be forthcoming.

But the use of Krebiozen was not to be deterred by mere facts—at least not for a while. The drug's backers shrieked that there was a conspiracy, that the American Medical Association and the American Cancer Society were colluding to keep Krebiozen off the market, either to delay the advent of effective cancer treatment or to force Ivy, Durovic, et al. to divvy up the profits expected. During all of the initial ballyhoo, Ivy cleverly had made no firm claims about the drug, and he now asked only for further study. The Chicago Medical Society was not fooled; in the next month it suspended Ivy for exploiting a "secret remedy."

As the political tremors caused by Krebiozen mounted, the University of Illinois was the first institution to be shaken. President George Stoddard appointed a research validation committee under the chairmanship of Dr. Warren Cole, director of the department of surgery. After a six-month study of the reports, further trials were recommended by the committee. These were to be carefully controlled and conducted on both animals and human beings, and the chemistry of Krebiozen was to be studied in detail. Ivy agreed to these conditions, but the brothers Durovic did not. Stoddard then ruled the university out of bounds for Krebiozen and was supported by his faculty. The highly political board of trustees proceeded to bounce Stoddard from the presidency.

Though the scientific community had abandoned further studies on Krebiozen after the 1951 report in the *Journal of the American Medical Association,* the Krebiozen Research Foundation, its diehard supporters, and curious private physicians continued to experiment. In the "Report on Krebiozen" published by the foundation in 1962, 3,300 physicians were documented as having treated 4,227 patients. Such a large number of customers is indeed impressive, but were they satisfied customers? Not likely. Considering the numbers, one may infer that 80 percent of the physicians who tried Krebiozen did so only on one patient; 92 percent treated no more than two. Since cancer patients are common enough, the logical conclusion is that one or two trials were enough to convince most doctors that the much-touted medicine was worthless.

Not surprisingly, however, the Krebiozen Research Foundation was able to find glowing success stories in the case records returned to it. Objective improvement was claimed, with decreased tumor size in 61 percent of brain and spinal cord lesions, 70 percent of brain metastases, and 48 percent of breast cancers. These results may sound striking, but a closer look at two specific cases calls their value into question.

Ivy kept a research record on a Mr. Taietti, an Argentinian with bladder cancer who received Krebiozen. Though Ivy never saw this man, he recorded verbal reports from Durovic. On February 19, 1959, the following was entered: "The patient has remained well and a recent cystoscopy revealed a normal bladder." In 1961, Ivy wrote, "Patient is well and active." Yet investigation by the U.S. Food and Drug Administration revealed that the 1959 and 1961 reports were complete fabrications: Mr. Taietti had died on July 12, 1955, of bladder cancer.

A breast cancer patient, Orme Moritz, read about Krebiozen and then refused any other form of treatment. She was accepted by the Krebiozen Research Foundation and received Krebiozen for several months in 1958. Records from the foundation show Mrs. Moritz's condition at that time was "early operable." The tumor doubled in size during the Krebiozen therapy, and finally, after almost a year's delay, Ivy and Durovic recommended a radical mastectomy. Ten months later the unfortunate woman died of widespread breast cancer.

From what they had seen and read, a few private physicians became suspicious. In 1952, one California doctor wrote to ask for Krebiozen for a patient who had had a "bilateral pneumonectomy," the removal of both lungs. Though this condition is incompatible with life, no questions were asked, and Krebiozen was sent with the customary request for $9.50 per vial. When no payment was forthcoming, the doctor was rebilled at monthly intervals until the FDA was notified.

As though to make assurance doubly sure, another doctor wrote to the Krebiozen Research Foundation in March, 1963. His patient, as his letter stated, had had a bilateral *total* pneumonectomy. Nonetheless, the foundation promptly forwarded eight ampoules of Krebiozen and a bill for seventy-six dollars.

Any ordinary pill or chemical concoction would certainly have been doomed in the face of the damaging data continually being made public. But Krebiozen had many powerful friends in both organized labor and Congress who clamored loudly for a "fair test." Acquiescing to this brouhaha, the prestigious National Cancer Institute communicated to the Krebiozen Research Foundation the conditions under which the NCI conducted all trials of new drugs and under which it would study Krebiozen:

1. There must be a scientific basis for believing that the material may possibly be of benefit to cancer patients.

2. There must be adequate preliminary study with laboratory animals to identify the nature and quantitative aspects of toxicity, to ensure a maximum opportunity of preventing harm to the patient.

3. The material must be described and standardized well enough to assure that a definite entity or a reproducible material is being tested.

To this list of conditions the Krebiozen Research Foundation replied, on October 3, 1960, with its own series of nonnegotiable demands that seemed more appropriate for a cease-fire and exchange of prisoners of war than for medical research:

> 1) All details of the design and administration and bases of evaluation of the double blind test shall meet with the approval of Dr. Andrew C. Ivy and the Krebiozen Research Foundation.

2) Such details, noted above to be worked out with the advice and participation of Dr. Andrew C. Ivy or his appointees, must assure that Dr. Ivy or his designated medical representatives, which he can appoint according to his judgment of the situation, will have free and continuing access at all times to observe the patients and their treatment, all records pertaining to their treatment as well as the right to record in the clinical files any disagreements or evaluation of the effect of Krebiozen in the patients or any other omissions or commissions.

3) Within eight weeks after conclusion of the clinical tests, the results of the evaluating committee shall be published by the *Journal of the American Medical Association*. If there is not unanimity of opinion then any difference of opinion among members of the evaluating committee shall be published in the same publication simultaneously. It is an explicit condition of our acceptance of the proposal that Dr. Andrew C. Ivy and/or his appointees shall be guaranteed a full publication of the observations and conclusions regarding this test in the same publications simultaneously with that of the evaluating committee members, so that if there is difference of opinion, the scientific community shall have the opportunity to study our views.

4) The *New York Post* shall be an observer of all negotiations for implementing [this] proposal and shall at the conclusion of the test report any or all differences of opinion, if any, regarding results. The *New York Post* also agrees to report at any time during the clinical test, upon the request of any party, any claims of deviation from the agreements made among the parties to the test.

The NCI clinical trial was never carried out.

Though Ivy and the Durovic brothers had made a considerable sum from the Krebiozen they had peddled on their own, the real financial bonanza would come if Krebiozen could be licensed by the FDA and sold like penicillin, rather than as an investigational substance. In 1954, a "New Drug Application" was filed, but licensure was denied since Krebiozen was ruled a biologic product. As such, it would need to be licensed by the Division of Biologic Standards of the U.S. Public Health Service, which required a proof of efficacy as well as of safety. Above all, the chemical identity of Krebiozen whould have to be established.

What was Krebiozen, anyway? Was it a magic drug capable of curing cancer, or simply a common, medicinally worthless substance? Even the compound's supporters were becoming more troubled by this question. In September, 1961, samples of material labeled as pure Krebiozen were reluctantly delivered to the National Cancer Institute. These samples were analyzed by the NCI, the FDA, and consultants from several universities. The result: Krebiozen was found to be creatine monohydrate, a normal constituent of muscle and a common laboratory chemical available for thirty cents per gram.

Wrong, all wrong, howled the Krebiozen Research Foundation. The FDA had misinterpreted the data, overlooked the important facts. Creatine monohydrate was just a contaminant in what had been labeled pure Krebiozen. Trace quantities of real Krebiozen were there. And to prove the point, Dr. Durovic offered to furnish pure Krebiozen for another government analysis at the rock-bottom wholesale price, $170,000 per gram.

But the FDA did not need more Krebiozen from Durovic. By 1964, a large number of dated ampoules had been analyzed by the most sophisticated chemical techniques. The best years for Krebiozen turned out to be late 1959 through 1963, when the ampoules proved to contain creatine or two other common chemicals, 1-methylhydantoin and amyl alcohol, dissolved in mineral oil. The years 1949 through early 1959 were not so good: all ampoules analyzed from this period contained nothing but mineral oil, and again after 1963 mineral oil was the only ingredient.

A full-scale FDA investigation of the case records of the

Krebiozen Research Foundation was then undertaken, and results agreed completely with the chemical tests. Of 4,307 records
of cancer patients treated before 1962, 2,781 were unacceptable
for evaluation because of overlapping treatments, lack of proof
of diagnosis, inadequate documentation, or lack of other standard prerequisites for judgment of therapeutic results in cancer.
However, 1,526 patients had records considered acceptable for
a determination of effect. Of these, three patients were found
in whom it was possible, but not certain, that partial regressions
of the tumor might have occurred. One remission was of two
weeks' duration; one remission was a reduction in size of a
primary breast cancer from which large biopsies had been taken
during therapy; and in the third, a 50 percent decrease in the
size of a lymph node three-quarters of an inch in diameter was
seen, though a coexistent cancer observed in the chest X ray was
never restudied. Of the other 1,523 patients, none received any
benefit from Krebiozen.

By the fall of 1963, the FDA was positive that Krebiozen
was worthless, but the agency had a problem deciding what
action to take. Its involvement began as an effort to help the
National Cancer Institute gather data on Krebiozen-treated patients but soon spread into an ambitious campaign to reconstruct all aspects of the drug's clinical, financial, and chemical
history. Past zeal to rout out quacks had hindered the FDA's
effort to maintain its scientific credibility, and now its reputation was definitely on the line. If Krebiozen were ever demonstrated to be something other than creatine, the agency, fighting
hard for a progressive image, would find itself aligned instead
with all the discredited reactionaries in the history of science.
So there seemed only two paths of action open: (1) go for
broke, or (2) forget the whole thing.

The government decided to go for broke. Ivy and the Durovics were to be treated as crooks rather than erring scientists,
their fate to be determined by a splashy criminal trial. In the
past, such a risky procedure had been entered upon only reluctantly, since the government would be barred from appealing

an adverse verdict. But Krebiozen was still available in Illinois, though shipment across state lines was prohibited, and FDA officials wanted all supply lines closed down permanently.

In October, 1964, the Justice Department went to a Chicago grand jury and obtained a massive forty-nine-count indictment charging conspiracy, mail fraud, mislabeling, and making false statements to the government. A conviction would put the directors of the Krebiozen Research Foundation into striped lab coats for over a hundred years and possibly force them to pay several hundred thousand dollars as well. In an unprecedented move, $500,000 bail was set for each of the Durovic brothers, though this was later disallowed by a judge, who released the two on their own recognizance. Nonetheless, the government had made its position on Ivy and the Durovics quite clear: these men were vicious desperadoes and should be treated as such. This was a fatal error.

When the trial began on April 29, 1965, the government based its case on a simple premise—too simple, as matters turned out. Krebiozen was a complete hoax. Durovic could not have produced his compound by the method he claimed, at the time he claimed, or in the amounts he claimed, the government said. Durovic's statement that Krebiozen could be produced for $170,000 per gram was false because, since Krebiozen was creatine, it would cost thirty cents a gram, and "even if Krebiozen could be produced by the method allegedly used . . . it would cost about $8,000 per gram. . . ."

Unfortunately for the government, demonstration that Krebiozen was creatine involved extensive, complex testimony on the chemistry of the compound. No member of the jury hearing this testimony had more than a high school education, and since the chemistry was intimately related with efficacy against cancer, the defense was quick to exploit emotions much more palpable to laymen than chemical formulae.

The Krebiozen Research Foundation lawyers kept the galleries full of those patients who believed themselves benefited by Krebiozen, probably members of that group of 2,781 cases with poor documentation. The jurors were, no doubt, deeply moved by the ardent testimonials from these former sufferers, just as Aimee Semple McPherson and Kathryn Kuhlman believers might have been. What did those government scientists with all their slick statistics know about a medicine that made sick folks feel better? "There was no proof that Krebiozen wasn't worth anything . . . we did not want to destroy Krebiozen," commented one juror to a Chicago newspaper after the trial.

Andrew Conway Ivy's reputation as a scientist also affected the jury. Though the government maintained that "an unusual activity in his bank account" in recent years explained his involvement with Krebiozen, Ivy testified that he had merely been lucky in the stock market. In the end, the distinguished, white-haired professor was most credible. "Ivy's reputation is known all over," remarked one juror after the trial. "I don't think a man would throw away fifty years of work for humanity and just dump it overboard."

When compared to the principal charges of conspiracy and mail fraud, some of the other charges—those that could be most well substantiated, unfortunately—seemed relatively petty: that the defendants violated laws governing investigational drugs by shipping Krebiozen across state borders without the experimental follow-up the law requires; that their motives were pure commercialization and not experimentation. Jurors remarked that they had been impressed by the government's evidence that the Durovics made money and wanted to convict them of something, but the charges of commercialization and fraud were so intertwined this could not be done.

Before returning a verdict of guilty, a federal jury is supposed to be convinced of guilt beyond a reasonable doubt. The defense was careful to seed the minds of the jurors with many such doubts. For example, the prosecution leaned heavily on its claim that Durovic never purchased enough ether or benzene to process horse blood in the way he contended he did. The defense argued that more of these solvents were bought than the government claimed, and that special laboratory equipment permitted the material to be reused. In the twenty-thousand-page record of the trial, thousands of such details were left hanging.

In his closing argument to the jury, government prosecutor Arthur Connelly read aloud the Andersen fairy tale "The Emperor's New Clothes," contending that this same fable was the story of Krebiozen:

> You have the story here of the two swindlers who come from Argentina. They said they had the secret stuff in a vial. They said they dissolved it in mineral oil so no one could see it, and they thought no one could find whether it was there by any other means.
>
> They met the emperor, the man who considers himself to be the greatest of all scientists; a man who considers his opinions beyond question, beyond question by anyone. He provided these two swindlers with the rooms, and the other trappings to put the scheme over. The emperor cast in his scientific reputation. Without it, not a nickel's worth of this stuff could have been sold.
>
> Almost from the very first, if not from the very first, the emperor knew, or must have known, that this stuff didn't exist.
>
> When the skeptical asked to see the secret powder, the swindlers and the emperor himself made excuses and charged that those who doubted were prejudiced and motivated by ideas of themselves taking the profit from the secret stuff.
>
> Then came the little boy, the Food and Drug Administration, who knew that if the stuff existed as the swindlers and the emperor claimed, that it at least ought to be visible in the amounts that they claimed it was in these ampoules. ... When finally the time came when the stuff could no longer be sheltered by excuses, claims, or unfairness, it turned out not to be beautiful, unique fabric at all. It was a common chemical and the shots offered as the greatest treatment for cancer were mineral oil.
>
> Even when presented with overwhelming scientific evidence, even when their own chemist identified the stuff

as creatine, the swindlers and the emperor persisted. Why?
In 1950–1951 because they hoped to sell the secret to
Abbott, or Lilly Laboratories for millions. For this they
falsified the results of clinical trials, as well as the truth
about the stuff.
From 1956 until today because mineral oil at prices from
$9.50 to $95.00 per ampoule was making them rich from
frantic cancer patients grasping for a straw of hope.

In the end, the government's clever fairy-tale analogy and
claim that Krebiozen and creatine were identical, both possessing
no anticancer activity, failed to impress the jury sufficiently.
The scientific conflicts were far beyond the capacity of a lay-
man to arbitrate, and the many hours of conflicting testimony
would have made any juror hesitate to vote for conviction. At
the close of the trial, even some members of the scientific community remained perplexed. Could Krebiozen have been a fraud
so flawless in its execution that it defied convincing exposure?
Or did it represent a scientific conflict so profound that no
tools were adequate to deal with it? Certainly the lay jurors
could not be expected to resolve these questions beyond a reasonable doubt; during eight days of deliberation they twice informed the judge of a hopeless deadlock. Finally, on January
30, 1966, Dr. Andrew Ivy, Marko Durovic, and one associate
were acquitted. On January 31, Dr. Stevan Durovic and the
Krebiozen Research Foundation were also found innocent.

At first the government took its defeat as a major disaster,
since many officials close to the case believed the government's
evidence complete and its conclusions logical. The verdict was
attributed to the emotionally charged issue and the popularity
of Ivy. "We were doomed from the beginning," one official
commented. "It wouldn't have made any difference what we said
or did."

For the Krebiozen forces, the world initially seemed brighter
after the trial. Ivy filed a $392,000 libel suit against his old
boss, George Stoddard, deposed president of the University of
Illinois. Several suits were filed on behalf of groups of patients

and individuals charging conspiracy on the part of the government, voluntary health agencies, and the American Medical Association to prevent interstate distribution of Krebiozen. But proponents of the notorious cancer cure soon found they were fighting a losing battle. Court after court ruled against them, and in 1973, an antiquackery ordinance passed by the Illinois legislature stopped the sale of Krebiozen in the last state where this had been legal.

Shortly after the Krebiozen trial's conclusion in 1966, Dr. Stevan Durovic was indicted for the evasion of $904,907 in income tax for the years 1960, 1961, and 1962. Government investigators had discovered that large sums of money had been withdrawn from bank accounts of Krebiozen's manufacturer, Promak Laboratory, and sent to Canadian and Swiss banks by Durovic. Unfortunately, the Internal Revenue Service was not sufficiently adroit to trap the wily Yugoslav.

During the trial, news of the impending tax evasion indictment somehow leaked to Durovic. When the government learned this, it attempted to watch the international airports so that escape from the country would be impossible. But Durovic managed to slip through the net, flying from Miami to Bimini in the Bahamas, from Bimini to Nassau, from Nassau to Bermuda, from Bermuda to London, from London to Paris, and from Paris to Switzerland.

Later questioned by reporters, Durovic stated that he did not owe the United States a penny and would return to Chicago to clear his good name after his treatment was over. It seems he had contracted tuberculosis and intended to take a long Alpine rest cure. Subsequently, one of Durovic's attorneys rather unsympathetically filed a suit seeking $11,787 in unpaid legal fees.

Though his former research partner had defected, the indefatigable Ivy continued to promote his anticancer substance, calling it by a new name, Carcalon. As late as 1972, Ivy was still said to be seeing patients in his Chicago office.

Krebiozen injections may today be obtained from Dr. Ernesto

Contreras in Tijuana, or from the Silbersee Clinic in Bonn, Germany. In the United States, Krebiozen is now dead as an issue—as dead as the unfortunate cancer victims who tried it—having ended its days in the ice of repeated clinical failures rather than in the fire of an emotional judicial proceeding.

Laetrile

In California, where so many health fads and cures originate, the drug Laetrile was born. A San Francisco physician, Dr. Ernst T. Krebs (1877–1970), cooked up the compound sometime before 1920, supposedly inspired by the so-called Beard Trophoblastic Theory of Cancer. One highlight of the Beard Theory: "Cancer is a chymotrypsin and nutritional deficiency disease, and . . . pancreatic chymotrypsin prevents about 80 percent of civilization from every developing malignancy, while in the other 20 percent, benign or malignant tumors will always arise, unless prevented by adequate screening tests and chemotherapy."

Krebs is reported to have extracted the first Laetrile samples from apricot kernels, later chemically characterizing his wondrous substance as laevo-mandelonitrile-beta-glucuronoside. The remedy was said to release cyanide "in the cancer areas, without injury to other tissue."

"Laetrile acts only upon cancer cells," said Krebs, "with the result that when all the cancer cells are destroyed there is still a tumor—but it is now benign." As soon as the "Beard Anthrone Test" was negative, "the surgeon should remove the benign growth." A maintenance dose of Laetrile was then supposed to be required for the remainder of the patient's life.

By 1953, the Cancer Commission of the California Medical Association had investigated Laetrile as a treatment for cancer in human beings. Its report in *California Medicine* concluded:

> The Commission had collected information concerning forty-four patients treated with Laetrile, all of whom either have active disease or are dead of their disease, with one exception. Of those alive with disease, no patient has been

found with objective evidence of control of cancer under treatment with Laetrile alone.

Nine patients dying from cancer after treatment with
Laetrile have been autopsied, and histological studies
done for the Commission by five different pathologists
have shown no evidence of any chemotherapeutic effect.

In two independent studies by experienced research
workers, Laetrile has been completely ineffective when
used in large doses on cancer in laboratory animals, in
lesions which are readily influenced in useful chemotherapy.

On May 15, 1965, the *Canadian Medical Association Journal*
published a report of an investigation of two forms of Laetrile:
"From the data obtained neither product can be considered as
a palliative in cancer therapy on the basis of the biological rationale advanced by the manufacturer."

As did the formulators of Krebiozen and other worthless
cancer remedies, the makers of Laetrile found a ready market
of cancer victims willing to try anything. To prevent such ex-
ploitation, the Food and Drug Administration brought suit in
the U.S. District Court of San Francisco in 1962. Ernst T.
Krebs, Jr., the doctor's son, and associates pled guilty to five
counts of violating new-drug provisions, and a fine of $3,755
was assessed. Krebs received a suspended prison sentence and
was placed on three years' probation with the specific provision
that he be prohibited from the interstate shipment of any new
drug, including Laetrile.

On August 2, 1965, Dr. Ernst T. Krebs agreed to a permanent court injunction against further distribution of Laetrile.
The eighty-seven-year-old physician told the U.S. District Court
in San Francisco that he was going out of the Laetrile business.
In September, 1965, he pleaded no contest to criminal contempt
charges stating he disobeyed a restraining order prohibiting shipment of Laetrile in interstate commerce. But like pornographers
and politicians, makers of worthless cancer remedies can flout
laws, and Laetrile continued to be sold and distributed throughout the United States.

On January 21, 1966, Dr. Krebs pleaded guilty to a contempt charge of shipping Laetrile in violation of an injunction. On February 3, 1966, he was given a suspended sentence of one year by a California U.S. District Court for failing to register as a producer of drugs, namely Laetrile. The judge indicated that he would impose a substantial fine if Dr. Krebs violated a permanent injunction against sales of Laetrile during his probation.

Laetrile distribution is now banned in Canada as well as the U.S., though a few state legislatures have contravened federal regulations and legalized the drug for intrastate use. The National Cancer Institute of Canada and the Canadian Medical Association think that the compound may even be harmful if used to treat cancer patients. To resolve this problem, Dr. Ernesto Contreras in Mexico and Dr. Hans Nieper in Germany, who are still using Laetrile, have been asked by the U.S. Food and Drug Administration to provide any records of treatment that they have.

But as of this moment, medical authorities are in agreement with the American Cancer Society, which states that it "does not have evidence that treatment with Laetrile results in objective benefit in the treatment of cancer in human beings."

The Grape Diet

This rather novel cancer cure was proposed by a Miss Johanna Brandt. Born in South Africa in 1876, Brandt claimed she fought a "nine year battle for life." After numerous fasts of varying length, she "accidentally discovered" that a diet consisting exclusively of grapes was a cure for cancer. After arriving in the United States in 1927, the studious Miss Brandt matriculated and spent six months in the postgraduate course of the First National University of Naturopathy of Newark, New Jersey. This august institution, allowing credit for unspecified previous work, awarded Brandt two degrees: Doctor of Naturopathy (N.D.) and Honorary Philosopher of Naturopathy (Ph.N.).

With kudos in hand, Brandt established herself in New York City, where she founded the Harmony Healing Centre. But alas, the centre was charged by unsympathetic state officials with practicing medicine without a license, and closed down. Soon afterward, one F. W. Collins, calling himself dean of the First National University of Naturopathy, Newark, New Jersey, announced that his institution had become the headquarters of the centre. Though no one is quite certain where Brandt or her centre are today, her legacy survives in the form of a classic cancer-cure book—*The Grape Cure.*

What is the grape diet? It consists of grape meal, which might vary from two ounces to half a pound of any good variety of grapes, taken starting at 8:00 A.M. and repeated every two hours. The book helpfully adds, "A loathing for grapes indicates the need for a fast. Skip a few meals." The rationale of treatment is: "The grape is highly antiseptic and a powerful solvent of inorganic matter deposits, fatty degeneration, morbid and malignant growths. It acts as a drastic eliminator of evil while building new tissue. . . ."

Though a deluge of adverse publicity at one time threatened to obliterate the grape diet, a resurgence in popularity of health foods and items sold in health food stores has sparked renewed interest. *The Grape Cure* is available in paperback in most health food stores, and recently articles promoting the grape cure have appeared in the magazines *Herald of Health* and *Prevention.* But the most authoritative and scientifically accurate appraisal of this remedy is that of the American Cancer Society: "After careful study of the literature and other available information, the American Cancer Society does not have evidence that treatment with the 'Grape Diet' results in objective benefit in the treatment of cancer in human beings."

The Gerson Treatment

Does a diet of green leaf juice and fresh calf's liver juice sound like a good cancer remedy? Dr. Max Gerson thought so, and he published his experience with this method in *A Cancer*

Therapy: Results of Fifty Cases, a 402-page book still in print. Gerson received his inspiration for this treatment while practicing internal medicine in Germany during the 1920s. A longtime sufferer from migraine headaches, the doctor one day discovered that nutritional therapy and adherence to a special diet helped lessen the attacks. This interesting observation had been made many times before, but not with Gerson's striking conclusion: since dietary therapy is good for headaches, it must be good for cancer, too.

Gerson left Germany in 1933, emigrated to the United States in 1936, and passed medical boards and became a U.S. citizen in 1942. He prospered in New York. His private office was located at 815 Park Avenue, and he managed to acquire a nursing home called Oakland Manor in Nanuet, New York, where he treated his patients; this institution was closed just prior to his death in April, 1959.

The Gerson Treatment received a big boost in 1947, when the noted author John Gunther brought his son for therapy. The boy, suffering from a recurrent, inoperable brain tumor, was given the full regimen: no foods except fresh fruits, vegetables, and oatmeal; no salt, spices, sodium bicarbonate, alcohol, or tobacco; milk proteins and supplemental vitamins A and D, niacin, and brewer's yeast; fresh, defatted bile in capsules; liver and iron capsules; dicalcium phosphate and viosterol; intramuscular injections of crude liver extract. The severe dehydration produced by the therapy and a delayed reaction from previous radiation and drug treatment led to a brief remission in the disease; this was duly described in Gunther's famous book *Death Be Not Proud.*

Gerson soon received another cancer victim on whom to try his treatment, a young boy brought by his parents after amputation had been advised for a bone tumor. After a prolonged stay at the nursing home and Gerson's ministrations, the child was returned home in a pathetic state of malnutrition and died a few days later.

As might be expected, accurate studies soon proved the Gerson Treatment to be worthless. Reports in the *Journal of the American Medical Association* in 1946 and 1949 concluded that the method was of no value. A 1947 review by the National Cancer Institute of ten cases selected by Gerson was no more promising. In the same year, a group appointed by the Committee on Cancer of the New York County Medical Society went over the records of eighty-six patients and examined ten patients. Again no scientific evidence could be found that supported Gerson's claims for the efficacy of his regimen. The doctor's malpractice insurance was subsequently discontinued in 1953, and on March 4, 1958, he was suspended for a period of two years from the New York Medical Society.

But the Gerson Method lives on, promoted by the widow, Mrs. Margaret Gerson, and three daughters. Interest has also been stimulated by numerous articles in such health magazines as *Prevention* and *Herald of Health*. The March/April 1972 issue of the *Cancer News Journal*, a publication of the International Association of Cancer Victims and Friends, Inc., depicts the "Gerson Cancer Therapy" on its cover. A more recent issue of the magazine helpfully indicated that more information could be obtained from Gerson's daughter, Mrs. Charlotte Straus, who lives in Queens, New York. But prudent cancer patients would do better to heed a source of medical information more reliable than a Queens housewife: "After a careful review of the literature and other information, the American Cancer Society does not have evidence that treatment of cancer in humans by the Gerson method results in any objective benefit."

16 In Brief

For the past fifty years, in spite of much fundamental and clinical research, radiation and surgery have continued to be the mainstays of cancer therapy. Drug therapy (chemotherapy) has made great strides in the past twenty years and can cure at least two formerly incurable cancers—choriocarcinoma of the uterus and acute lymphoblastic leukemia in childhood. But drug therapy is not presently competitive with radiation or surgery.

Yet many patients, and doctors, are not aware that though radiation and surgery can both be used in cancer treatment, radical radiotherapy and certain conservative surgical techniques may produce as many cures as the older, more radical surgical methods, preserving body function and appearance at the same time. These techniques are especially applicable to the following forms of cancer:

1. Breast cancer: lumpectomy (removal of tumor mass alone) and radiotherapy or radiotherapy alone appear to be as effective as radical mastectomy.
2. Tongue cancer and oral cancer: radical radiotherapy can produce cures without loss of tongue and larynx function.
3. Larynx cancer: radiation therapy is often curative, and the larynx is preserved.
4. Rectal cancer: local radiotherapy or fulguration (burning) and external radiotherapy can cure many lesions that would necessitate a colostomy if treated by older, radical surgical techniques.

5. Prostate cancer: radical radiotherapy is as effective as surgery and also preserves potency, which is inevitably lost after radical surgery.

A final problem: when a patient is cured of cancer, he or she often is discriminated against on the job. Though employment in the United States may not be denied on the basis of race, sex, or national origin, rejection of an applicant with a cancer history is widely practiced—even by our largest corporations. For this reason, a federal law is urgently needed forbidding job discrimination against cancer victims. Of what good are even the most sophisticated and effective forms of treatment if the cured patient cannot regain his place in society? Compassion and a sense of human decency demand nothing less.

Bibliography

1 The Cancer Problem

Ackerman, Lauren, and del Regato, Juan A. *Cancer.* The C. V. Mosby Company, 1970.

American Cancer Society Information Service. "What Real Progress Is Being Made Against Cancer?" 2, no. 2 (Spring/Summer 1975).

"Animal Study Shows Intriguing Link Between Chronic Stress, Cancer." *Journal of the American Medical Association* 233 (1975): 757–58.

"Cancer Facts and Figures." New York: American Cancer Society, 1975.

Rapp, Fred, and Westmoreland, Diana. "Do Viruses Cause Cancer in Man?" *CA* 25 (1975): 215–29.

Rubin, Philip, ed. *Clinical Oncology for Physicians and Medical Students.* New York: American Cancer Society, 1974.

2 Breast Cancer

Ackerman and del Regato. *Cancer.* Pp. 830–95.

Guttmann, Ruth. "Radiotherapy in Locally Advanced Cancer of the Breast." *Cancer* 20 (1967): 1046–50.

"Many Surgeons Prefer Old Methods of Treating Breast Cancer." *Journal of the American Medical Association* 234 (1975): 259.

Prosnitz, Leonard R., and Goldenberg, Ira S. "Radiation Therapy as Primary Treatment for Early Stage Carcinoma of the Breast." *Cancer* 35 (1975): 1587–96.

Rubin, *Clinical Oncology.* Pp. 129–49.

Weber, Eric, and Hellman, Samuel. "Radiation as Primary Treatment for Local Control of Breast Carcinoma." *Journal of the American Medical Association* 234 (1975): 608–11.

3 Lung Cancer

Ackerman and del Regato. *Cancer.* Pp. 329–76.
Beattie, Edward J., Jr. "Lung Cancer." *CA* 24 (1974): 96–99.
Rubin. *Clinical Oncology.* Pp. 150–63.

4 Cancer of the Female Reproductive Organs

Ackerman and del Regato. *Cancer.* Pp. 713–829.
Arje, Sidney L., and Hodgkinson, C. Paul. "The Current Status of Ovarian Cancer Control." *CA* 21 (1971): 365–67.
Gusberg, S. B. "An Approach to the Control of Carcinoma of the Endometrium." *CA* 23 (1973): 99–105.
Kaufman, Raymond H., and Rawls, William E. "Herpes Genitalis and Its Relationship to Cervical Cancer." *CA* 24 (1974): 258–65.
Koss, Leopold G. "Precancerous Lesions of the Uterine Cervix in Pregnancy." *CA* 24 (1974): 141–43.
Rubin. *Clinical Oncology.* Pp. 216–57.
Weigensberg, I. J. "Preoperative Therapy in Endometrial Carcinoma: Preliminary Report of a Clinical Trial." *American Journal of Roentgenology* 127 (1976): 319–23.

5 Cancer of the Digestive Tract

Ackerman and del Regato. *Cancer.* Pp. 408–605.
Crile, George. "Changing Concepts in the Management of Cancer." *Proceedings of the Royal Society, Medicine* 66 (1973): 1190.
"How Not to Die of Cancer." *Time,* May 10, 1963.
Lehrer, Steven. "Rectal Self-Examination." *American Journal of Digestive Diseases,* 23 (1978): 572–73.
"Liver Tumors and the Pill." *British Medical Journal,* 6 July 1974, 3–4.
Papillon, Jean. "Endocavitary Irradiation of Early Rectal Cancers for Cure: A Series of 123 Cases." *Proceedings of the Royal Society, Medicine* 66 (1973): 1179–81.

Pearson, James G. "Cancer of the Gastrointestinal Tract. II. Esophagus: Treatment—Localized and Advanced. Value of Radiation Therapy." *Journal of the American Medical Association* 227 (1974): 181–83.

"Regular Screening Would Reduce Cancer of the Colon and Rectum Toll." *Journal of the American Medical Association* 234 (1975): 137.

Roswit, Bernard; Higgins, G. A.; and Keehn, R. "Preoperative Irradation for Carcinoma of the Rectum and Rectosigmoid Colon: Report of a National Veterans Administration Randomized Study." *Cancer* 35 (1975): 1597–1602.

Rubin. *Clinical Oncology.* Pp. 198–215.

"Vinyl Chloride and Cancer." *British Medical Journal,* 30 March 1974, pp. 590–91.

6 Cancer of the Male Genital Tract and Urinary Tract

Ackerman and del Regato. *Cancer.* Pp. 606–82.

Bagshaw, M. A. "Definitive Radiotherapy in Carcinoma of the Prostate." *Journal of the American Medical Association* 210 (1969): 326–27.

Rubin. *Clinical Oncology.* Pp. 258–89.

7 Skin Cancer

Ackerman and del Regato. *Cancer,* Pp. 120–62.

L'Etang, Hugh. *The Pathology of Leadership.* Hawthorn Press, 1970. P. 95.

Rubin. *Clinical Oncology.* Pp. 258–89.

Schickel, Richard. "Doug Fairbanks: Superstar of the Silents." *American Heritage* (Dec 71): 4–12, 92–99.

8 Leukemias and Lymphomas

Ackerman and del Regato. *Cancer.* Pp. 978–1019.

Golde, D. W., and Cline, M. J. "Human Preleukemia: Identification of a Maturation Defect *in vitro." New England Journal of Medicine* 288 (1973): 1083.

Howell, Milton M. "The Lone Eagle's Last Flight." *Journal of the American Medical Association* 232 (1975): 715.

Penn, I. "Malignant Tumors Arising de Novo in Immunosupressive Organ Transplant Recipients." *Transplantation* 14 (1972): 407–17.
Rubin. *Clinical Oncology.* Pp. 425–87.
"Rudolf Virchow." *CA* 25 (1975): 91–92.
"Sidney Farber." *CA* 24 (1974): 294–96.
"Thomas Hodgkin." *CA* 23 (1973): 52–53.

9   Tumors of the Nervous System

Courtney, J. F. "Doctors and George Gershwin." *Resident and Staff Physician,* December 1969, pp. 55–58.
Fabricant, Noah. *Thirteen Famous Patients.* Philadelphia: Chilton Co., 1960. Pp. 193–201.
Metz, Robert. "The Biggest Man in Broadcasting." *New York,* July 21, 1975, p. 44.
Rubin. *Clinical Oncology.* Pp. 343–58.

10   Tumors of the Eye

Ackerman and del Regato. *Cancer.* Pp. 956–77.
Rubin, Philip. *Clinical Oncology.* Pp. 359–76.

11   Tumors of the Head and Neck

Ackerman and del Regato. *Cancer.* Pp. 163–328.
Aronson, Theo. "Empress Victoria." *Horizon* 16 (1974): 102–5.
Bettmann, Otto L. *A Pictorial History of Medicine.* Springfield, Ill.: C. C. Thomas, 1956. P. 267.
Fabricant. *Thirteen Famous Patients.* Pp. 157–68.
Jones, Ernest. *The Life and Work of Sigmund Freud. The Last Phase 1919–1939.* New York: Basic Books, 1957. Pp. 119–248.
Lott, S.; El Mahdi, A. M.; and Hazra, T. "Supervoltage Radiotherapy for Carcinoma of the Larynx. The Johns Hopkins Hospital Results 1961–1967." *Johns Hopkins Journal of Medicine* 130 (1972): 244–53.
Marx, Rudolf. *The Health of the Presidents.* New York: Putnam, 1961. Pp. 205–19, 253–62.
Rubin. *Clinical Oncology.* Pp. 303–42.

12   Tumors of Bone and Soft Tissue

Ackerman and del Regato. *Cancer.* Pp. 896–955.
Rubin. *Clinical Oncology.* Pp. 377–404.
"Teddy's Ordeal." *Time,* Dec 3, 1973, p. 86.

13   Tumors of Children

Ackerman and del Regato. *Cancer.* Pp. 607–24, 691–708, 956–74.
Chatlen, J., and Voorhess, M. L. "Familial Neuroblastoma." *New England Journal of Medicine* 227 (1967): 1230.
Rubin. *Clinical Oncology.* Pp. 487–507.

14   Tumors of the Thyroid and Adrenal Glands

Ackerman and del Regato. *Cancer.* Pp. 377–95, 691–712.
Rubin. *Clinical Oncology.* Pp. 405–24.

15   Cancer and Baloney: Management Methods of Dubious Value

"The Gerson Method." *CA* 23 (1973): 314–17.
"The Grape Diet." *CA* 24 (1974): 144–46.
Holland, James F. "The Krebiozen Story. Is Cancer Quackery Dead?" *Journal of the American Medical Association* 200 (1967): 125–30.
Holleb, Arthur I. "Worthless Cancer Remedies." *CA* 21 (1971): 71.
"The Krebiozen Affair." *New England Journal of Medicine* 269 (1963): 531–32.
"Krebiozen and Carcalon." *CA* 23 (1973): 111–15.
"Laetrile." *CA* 22 (1972): 245–51.
Langer, Eleanor. "The Krebiozen Case: What Happened in Chicago." *Science* 151 (1966): 1061–64.

Index

Acromegaly, 107
Actinomyces bovis, 152
Actinomycin D, 90, 139
Acute lymphocytic leukemia, 88–92
Acute myelogenous leukemia, 87–88
Addison, Thomas, 146
Addison's disease, 146–49
"Addison's pill," 146
Adenocarcinoma, 25, 44, 70, 76
Adenomatoris hyperplasia, 38
Adenosarcoma, 9
Adrenal cortex, 147
Adrenal glands, 146–49
Age factor in cancer, 2–3
Aldosterone, 147
American Cancer Society, 50, 155, 168, 169; Reach to Recovery, 21
American Chemical Society, 86
American College of Surgeons, 12, 19
American Medical Association, 155, 165
Aminopterin, 89
Anaplastic carcinoma, 145
Androgen, 147
Anemia, 51–52
Angiogram, 108, 148
Angiosarcoma, 64
Aniline, 5
Antibodies, 32

Arrhenoblastoma, 41
Asbestos dust, 5
Astrocytoma, 106
Autosomal dominance, 4

Bagshaw, Malcolm, 71
Bantu people, 1–2, 54, 63
Basal cell carcinomas, 81
Basophilic adenoma, 106
BCG vaccine, 83–84, 92
Beard Trophoblastic Theory of Cancer, 166
Bence-Jones protein, 8, 100
Bennett, John Hughes, 85
Benzidine, 5
Bergerac, Michael, 62
Beta-napthylamine, 5
B. F. Goodrich Company, 64
Bile ducts, cancer of, 66–67
Billroth, Theodore, 53
Billroth II operation, 53
Biopsy, 33–34, 65, 81
Bloody menopause, 37
Body development, precocious, 76
Bone cancers, 131–33
Bone infection, 81
Bone marrow transplant, 92
Bowel cancer, 54–61
Brady, Diamond Jim, 70
Brady Urologic Institute, 70
Brain tumors, 108
Brandt, Johanna, 168–71
Breast cancer, 4–5, 13–21, 173

Bronchoscopy, 26
Burkitt's lymphoma, 98
Busulfan, 88

California Medical Association
Cancer Commission, 166–67
California Medicine, 166
Canadian Medical Association, 168
*Canadian Medical Association
Journal,* 167
Cancer: adrenal glands, 146–49;
bone, 131–33; bowel, 54–61;
breast, 4–5, 13–21, 173;
cells, 8–9; central nervous
system, 103–9; cervical,
31–36; checkups, 11; in
children, 137–42; cure and
survival rate, 10–11; danger
signals, 11; eye, 111–12,
137–39; endometrium, 37;
esophagus, 47–50; gall
bladder/bile ducts, 66–67;
head and neck, 113–29;
heredity factor, 3–4, 86–87;
kidney, 76–78, 139–40;
larynx, 120–24, 173;
leukemias, 85–93; lips, 127;
liver, 63–66, 142; lung,
23–29; male genital and
urinary tract, 69–78;
mastectomies, 18–19; muscle,
142; nasal fossa, 126–27;
nasopharynx, 126–27; nervous
system, 140–41; ovaries,
40–42; palate, 115–20;
pancreas, 61–63; paranasal
sinuses, 125–26; penis, 78;
possible causes, 4–7;
prostate gland, 69–72, 173;
radiation therapy, 20; racial
factors, 1–2, 11, 47, 78, 80,
82, 83; rectal, 173; salivary
glands, 127; sex factor, 2;
skin, 79–84; soft tissue,
134–35; stomach, 50–53;
testicles, 75–76; therapies,
173–74; thyroid, 143–46;
tongue, 113–15, 173; types of,
9–10, 52–53, 81–4, 145;
urinary bladder, 72–75; uterus,
36–40, 44–45; vagina, 44;
viruses, 3; vulva, 42–44
*Cancer Therapy: Results of Fifty
Cases* (Gerson), 169–70
Cancer News Journal, 171
Carcinoembryonic antigen
(CEA), 56
Carcinogenic agents, 5–6, 24
Carcinoma, 9; breast and uterus,
2–3
Cataract, radiation, 138
Cavanaugh, Patrick, 63
Cellular Pathology (Virchow), 85
Central nervous system, 103–9
Cervical cancers, stages of, 35
Cervix, 31–36
Chatlen, J., 140
Chemical trauma, 5
Chemotherapy, 97, 109
Chest X rays, 25, 28
Chicago Medical Society, 155
Children, cancer in, 137–42
Chlorambucil, 42
Chloramphenical, 86
Chondrosarcoma, 133
Choriocarcinoma, 76; of the
uterus, 44–45
Chorionic gonadotropin, 45
Chrome salts, 5
Chronic lymphocytic leukemia,
92–93
Chronic myelogenous leukemia, 88
Chronic psychic stress, 4
Church, Frank, 76
Cigarette smoking, 24, 73
Cirrhosis of the liver, 63–66
Cleveland, Grover, 125
Clonorchis sinensis, 64
Cole, Warren, 155
Collins, F. W., 169
Colon, cancer of the, 54–61
Colonoscope, 56
Colostomy, 57
Colposcopy, 34
Computerized axial tomographic
scanner, 63, 77, 108, 139

Concerto in F (Gershwin), 103,
    104
Connelly, Arthur, quoted, 163–64
Contact inhibition, 8
Contreras, Ernesto, 165–66, 168
Cortisone, 109
Courtial, J., 78
Craniopharyngioma, 107
Crile, George, Jr., 58
"Criteria of inoperability," 18
Cure rates of cancer, 10–11
Curie, Marie, 14
Cushing, Harvey, 106
Cushing's disease, 106; syndrone,
    147
Cystectomy, 74
Cystic glandular hyperplasia, 38
Cystic and noncystic ovary
    cancer, 40–41
Cytoxan, 42
Czermak, Johann, 121

D & C (dilatation and curettage),
    34, 37
Dandy, Walter, 105, 108
Death Be Not Proud (Gunther),
    170
Deutsch, Felix, 117
Diabetes insipidus, 107
Disease as cancer cause, 6
Disney, Walt, 23
DNA, 7
DNCB cream, 82
Down's syndrome, 86–87
Drugs, anticancer, 28, 42, 45, 65,
    82, 89–91, 138
Duke Medical School, 63
Durovic, Marko, 152, 164
Durovic, Stevan, 152–65
Dysphagia, 48

Edinburgh, Scotland, 50
Embryonal carcinoma, 76
Endometrial hyperplasia, 38
Ependymoma, 106
Epidermoid carcinomas, 10, 33
Epinephrine, 140, 147, 148
Erb's palsy, 122

Erdheim, Jacob, 119
Erythroleukemia, 86
Esophagus, 47–50
Estrogen, 147
Estrogen U, 72
Ewing, James, quoted, 11–12
Ewing's sarcoma, 133
Eye tumors, 111–12, 137–39

Facial asymmetry, 138
Fairbanks, Douglas, 80
Familial polyposis of the colon, 55
Farber, Sydney, 89, 139, 140
Fasciola hepatica, 64
Fiberoptic duodenoscope, 62
Fibrocystic disease, 16–17
Fibrosarcoma, 9, 134
Finland, 50, 54
First National University of
    Naturopathy, 169
Flexible gastroscope, 52
5-Fluorouracil, 42, 65
Follicuar carcinoma, 145
Franconi's anemia, 87
Freud, Sigmund, 115–20

Gallbladder and bile ducts, 6,
    66–67
Gallstones, 6
Ganglioneuroma, 148
Garcia, Manuel, 121, 123
Gastric polyps, 51
Gerhardt, Karl, 121
Gershwin, George, 103–5
Gerson, Margaret, 171
Gerson, Max, 169–71
Gerson treatment, 169–71
Glioblastoma multiform, 106
Glioma, 105–6
Globus hystericus, 48
Golde, D. W., 92
Gone with the Wind, 79
Graham, Evarts, 27
Granular cell myoblastoma, 43
Granulosa-theca cell tumors, 41
Grant, Ulyses, S., 114
Grape diet, 168–69
Grape Diet (Brandt), 169

Growths, noncancerous, 16–17
Gunther, John, 170
Guttman, Ruth, 19

Hajek, Marcus, 116
Halsted, William S., 14
Hana, Hawaii, 99
Harmony Healing Center, 169
Haslam, John, 63
Hematuria, 77
Hemochromatosis, 64
Hepatoma, 142
Herald of Health, 169, 171
Heredity factor in cancer, 3–4, 86–87
Herpeslike virus, 98
Herpesvirus type two, 32
Herta, R., 45
Hindus, 5
Hodgkin, Thomas, 93–94
Hodgkin's disease, 93–97
Holleb, Arthur, 151
Hormonal therapy of prostate cancer, 72
Hormones, 20
Hounsfield, Godfrey, 108
Huggins, Charles, 72
Hydatidiform mole, 45
Hypernephroma, 76
Hysterectomy, 35, 38

Iceland, 2, 50
Institutio Biologica Duga (Buenos Aires), 152
Interstitial cell tumor, 76
Intraocular melanoma, 112
Intravenous pyelogram, 74, 76, 77, 148
Ivory Soap, 59
Ivy, Andrew C., 152–65

Japan, 50, 54
Jewett, Hugh, 73
Jewish women, breast cancer among, 15
Johns Hopkins Hospital, 28
Jones, Ernest, quoted, 115–17
Journal of the American Medical Association, 75, 154, 155, 158, 171

Kaplan, Henry, 96
Kaposi's hemorrhagic sarcoma, 1–2, 82–83
Kennedy, Edward M., 132
Kennedy, Edward M., Jr., 131–33
Kennedy, Joan, 132
Kennedy, John F., 147
Kidneys, 76–78, 139–40
Klinefeller's syndrome, 87
Kositerin, 152,
Krasno, Louis R., 153
Krebiozen controversy, 152–64
Krebiozen Research Foundation, 156–61
Krebs, Ernst T., 166–68
Krebs, Ernst T., Jr., 167
Kuhlman, Kathryn, 162
Kurland, L. T., 103
KY Lubricating Jelly, 59

La Brosse Spot Test, 141
Laetrile, 166–68
Large bowel, 54–59
Laryngoscope, 121, 123–24
Larynx, 120–24, 173
L'Etang, Hugh, 84
Leukemia, 5, 7, 85–93
Leukoplakia, 6, 43, 127
Leydig cells, 76
Lindbergh, Anne Morrow, 99
Lindbergh, Charles, 98–100
Liposarcoma, 134
Lips, cancer of the, 127
Liver, 1, 5, 63–66, 142
Liver scan, 65
Lobectomy, 27
Los Angeles Tumor Institute, 58
Lott, Steward, 124
L-phenylalanine mustard (L-PAM), 20
Lukes classification of Hodgkin cells, 95–96
Lumpectomy treatment, 18, 19
Lung cancer, 5, 10, 25
Lymphangiosarcoma, 134
Lymphatic tissue, 85–86
Lymphocytic leukemia, 86, 88–92
Lymphomas, 93–102

McGee, Frank, 100–101

Mackenzie, Morrell, 121–22
McPherson, Aimee Semple, 162
Madden, John, 59
Maimonides Medical Center, 135
Malignancy, degrees of, 9
Malignant melanoma, 2, 82, 83, 84, 111
Mammography, 16
Massie, F. M., 84
Mast cell leukemia, 86
Mastectomy: radical, 14, 18–19; simple, 18–19
Mayo Clinic, 28
Mediastenoscopy, 26–27
Medullary carcinoma, 145
Medulloblastoma, 107
Meland, Orville, 58
Melanoma, 111–12
Mendel, Gregor, 4
Mendelian dominance, 55
Meningioma, 106
6-mercaptopurine, 91
Metastasis, 8
Methotrexate, 45, 65, 89–90, 91, 133
Miles operation, 57, 58–59
Miller, Roscoe, 152
Minot, George, 51
Monocytic leukemia, 86
Mongolism, 86–87
MOPP regimen, 97
Moritz, Orme, 157
Morow, Dwight, 99
Multiple myeloma, 7–8, 100–101
Multiple-step induction theory, 7
Murphy, William, 51
Muscle tumor, 142
Mustard gas, 90
Mycosis fungoides, 82
Myelogenous leukemia, 86, 87–88
Myelogenous tissues, 85–86
Myelography, 108

Naffziger, Howard, 105
Nasal fossa, 126–27
Nasopharynx, 126–27
National Cancer Institute, 11, 157, 158, 159, 171; Conference on Breast Cancer, 20

National Cancer Institute of Canada, 168
Neural crest tissue, 140
Neuroblastoma, 140–41
Neurohypophysis, 107
Nervous system, 140–141
New England Journal of Medicine, 92, 140
New Haven, Conn., 24
New York City's Memorial Hospital, 28
New York County Medical Society, 171
New York Post, 158
Nickel carbonyl, 5
Nieper, Hans, 168
Nitrogen mustard, 82, 90
Non-Hodgkin's lymphoma, 97–100
Norepinephrine, 141, 147, 148
Nucleation, 112

Oat cells, 25
O'Hara, Scarlett, 79–80
Orcovin, 97
Orthovoltage (250KEV radiation), 27
Osteogenic sarcoma, 133
Osteomyelitis, chronic, 81
Ovaries, 40–42

Paget's disease, 131
Palate, 115–20
Palliation, 27
Palpation test, 16
Pancreatic cancer, 61–63
Papanicolaou (Pap) test, 33, 37
Papillary carcinoma, 145, 146
Papilloma, 74
Papillon, Jean, 59
Pathology of Leadership (L'Etang), 84
Penis, 78
Penn, I., 98
Pernicious anemia, 51–52
Phenylalanine Mustard, 42
Phenylbutazone, 86
Pheochromocytoma, 148
Philadelphia chromosome, 88
Phillips, William F., 154
Phosphorous-22, 112

Index

185

Physical trauma, 5
Pichler, Hans, 117
Pick, John F., 154
Plasmacytic leukemia, 86
Plummer-Vinson syndrome, 47
Porgy and Bess (Gershwin), 104
Pott, Pervical, 81
Powell, William, 57–58, 59
Pneumonectomy, 27
Pneumoencephalogram, 108
Prednisone, 91, 97
Pregnancy: cervical cancer
during, 35–36; Hodgkin's
disease during, 97
Preleukemia, 92
Prevention, 169, 171
Princess Margaret Hospital
(Toronto), 57
Procarbazine, 97
Progesterone therapy, 39–40
Promak Laboratory, 165
Prosnitz, Leonard R., 19
Prostate cancer, 69–72, 173
Proteins, abnormal, 7–8
Prout, George, 75

Race factor in cancer, 1–2, 11,
47, 78, 80, 82, 83
Radiation treatment, 6, 14–15, 20,
27, 36, 38–39, 42, 44, 49, 53,
57, 63, 72, 74–75, 91–92, 100,
112, 114, 124, 133, 135,
143–44
Radical mastectomy, 14, 18–19
Radical prostatectomy, 71
Radical vulvectomy, 43
Radioactive iodine, 144
Radioisotope imaging, 17
Radiotherapy, 12
Radium, 6
Radon, A., 108
Raffla, S., 57
Rand, Carl, 104
Rayburn, Sam, 69, 70
Rectal cancer, 173
Rectal self-examination, 59–61
Rectilinear scanner, 65
Reed Sternberg cell, 95
Reese, A. B., 138

"Report on Krebiozen," 155
Rescue therapy, 133
Retinoblastoma, 2, 4, 111, 137–39
Retroperitoneal pneumography,
148
Revson, Charles, 61–62
Rhabdomyosarcoma, 134, 142
Rhapsody in Blue (Gershwin), 104
Rider, W., 57
Riley, Vernon, 4
Roentgen, Wilhelm, 14
Roosevelt, Franklin D., 84
Rosvit, Bernard, 57, 69

Salivary glands, 127–29
Sarcoma, 9
Sauerbray, R., 53
Scalene node biopsy, 26
Schiller test, 34
Schistosma hemalobrium, 73
Science, 4
Selective renal arteriogram, 77
Seminoma, 76
Sertoli-leydig cell tumor, 41
Sex factor in cancer, 2
Sigmoidoscope, 55, 56
Silbersee Clinic (Bonn, W.
Germany), 166
Simple mastectomy, 18–19
Sinuses, paranasal, 125–26
Sischy, Ben, 59
Skin cancer, 79–84
Small bowel, 54
Smallens, Alexander, 103
Smoking, 24, 73
Soft tissue, 134–35
South Carolina, 53
Spinal cord tumors, 108
Spinal tap, 108
Sputum cytology test, 26
Squamous cells, 25, 81
Stage zero cervical cancer, 34–35
"Status Report on Krebiozen," 154
Stoddard, George, 155, 164
Stomach cancer, 10, 50–53
Straus, Charlotte, 171
Stress, chronic psychic, 4
Sullivan, Ed. 47
Suntan craze, 80

Supervoltage radiation, 27
Surgery, 12, 43, 49, 53, 77, 108–9,
    133, 135, 141
Syphilis of the tongue, 6
Syringocystadenoma
    papilliferum, 43

Taietti, Mr., 156
Taihefer, A., 78
Tasaday people, 99
Technetrium 99m, 65;
    diphosphonate, 17;
    pertechnatate, 17;
    sulfacolloid, 17
TEM drugs, 138
Teratoma, 76, 142
Testicle cancer, 2, 75–76
Testosterone, 41
Thermography, 16
Thyroid gland, 143–46
Thyroid-stimulating hormone,
    143, 144
Time, quoted, 58–59, 131–32
Tongue cancer, 113–15, 173
Transplantation, 98
Tumors: adrenal glands, 146–49;
    in children, 137–42; eye,
    111–12; head and neck,
    113–29; nervous system,
    103–9; thyroid, 143–46
Türck, Ludwig, 121

Ulcerative colitis, 55
United States: Food and Drug
    Administration (FDA), 157,
    158, 159–61, 163, 167, 168;
    Justice Department, 161;
    Public Health Service's
    Division of Biologic
    Standards, 159
Upper gastrointestinal series of
    X-ray, 52

Urinary bladder cancer, 72–75
Uterine polyps, 37
Uterus, 7, 36–40, 44–45

Vagina, 44
Vanillomandelic acid. See VMA
    compound
Vaseline, 59
Veterans Administration hospitals,
    57
Venereal disease, 33
Victoria, Queen, 122
Vincristine, 91, 97
Vinyl chloride, 5
Virchow, Rudolf, 85
Viruses, 3
Vitamin B-12, 51
VMA compound, 141, 148
Von Recklinghausen's disease, 134
Vulva, 42–44

Waldenstrom's
    Macroglobulinemia, 101–2
Wallace, Lurleen, 31
Walter Reed Army Hospital, 84
Wayne, John, 23
Weber, Eric, 19
Wellman, William, 86
Whipple, George, 51
Whipple procedure, 63
Wilhelm, Kaiser, 122, 123
Wilhelm, Prince Friedrich, 121–24
Wilks, Samuel, 93
Wilm's tumor, 2, 90, 139–40

Xerodema pigmentosum, 3–4
Xeromammography, 16
X-rays, 6, 14, 48, 52, 56, 108

Young, Hugh Hampton, 70, 71

Zollinger-Ellison tumors, 62, 63